Understanding Atrial Fibrillation

Understanding Atrial Fibrillation

Peter Spector, MD

Professor of Medicine
Professor of Electrical and Biomedical Engineering
Director of Cardiac Electrophysiology and Cardiac Electrophysiology Laboratory
University of Vermont Medical Center
Burlington, VT, USA

WILEY Blackwell

Registered Office(s)
John Wiley & Sons, Inc., 111 River Street, Hoboken, NJ 07030, USA
John Wiley & Sons Ltd, The Atrium, Southern Gate, Chichester, West Sussex, PO19 8SQ, UK

Editorial Office
9600 Garsington Road, Oxford, OX4 2DQ, UK

For details of our global editorial offices, customer services, and more information about Wiley products visit us at www.wiley.com.

Wiley also publishes its books in a variety of electronic formats and by print-on-demand. Some content that appears in standard print versions of this book may not be available in other formats.

Library of Congress Cataloging-in-Publication Data

Names: Spector, Peter, author.
Title: Understanding atrial fibrillation / Peter Spector.
Description: Hoboken, NJ : Wiley-Blackwell, 2020. | Includes bibliographical
   references and index. |
Identifiers: LCCN 2019015123 (print) | LCCN 2019015570 (ebook) | ISBN 9781119524618
   (Adobe PDF) | ISBN 9781119524625 (ePub) | ISBN 9781119524601 (paperback)
Subjects: | MESH: Atrial Fibrillation–physiopathology | Atrial Fibrillation–diagnosis |
   Electrophysiologic Techniques, Cardiac–methods | Cardiac Electrophysiology–methods |
   Models, Cardiovascular
Classification: LCC RC685.A72 (ebook) | LCC RC685.A72 (print) | NLM WG 330.5.A5 |
   DDC 616.1/28–dc23
LC record available at https://lccn.loc.gov/2019015123

Cover Design: Wiley
Cover Image: © Peter S. Spector

Set in 10.5/13.5pt Minion Pro by SPi Global, Pondicherry, India
Printed and bound in Singapore by Markono Print Media Pte Ltd

10 9 8 7 6 5 4 3 2 1

"The history of the recognition of fibrillation of the auricles will impress you with the dimness of our eyes and the opacity of the obstacles which embarrass our vision. You will know how blind we have been to things which, once seen, are so apparent."

Thomas Lewis, MD, 1912

Contents

Preface

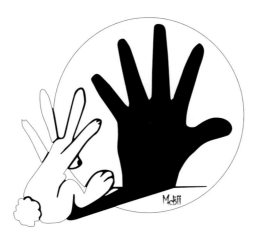

Why do we need another book about atrial fibrillation?

Despite the numerous good books available on the topic, there are several reasons I think it is worthwhile writing yet another book about atrial fibrillation (AF). Fibrillation involves elegant physiology that is not widely taught or understood, and as a result there are widespread misconceptions or ill-conceived beliefs about AF. Electrophysiology (EP) in general is an aesthetically attractive intellectual endeavor: it makes sense and lends itself well to deductive reasoning. If you think about the fundamental principles of EP, you can figure out most things, with no need for rote memorization. AF takes this deductive

Illustration: © Donald Brand

process to extremes: "if this is true, then that must be true," ad nauseam. We start by thinking about propagation in waves that traverse the tissue. Next, we think about more than one wave propagating at the same time, and consider how they interact. The outcome of such interactions is widely varied and depends in large part upon the timing and location of wave collisions. In AF there are numerous waves, traveling in random directions at random intervals, and hence the "space of possible interactions" is perpetually scanned; everything that can happen does happen. This roiling, random, and chaotic activation seems inscrutable and unpredictable. However, as we will see in this book, the immense complexity of activation during AF becomes tractable via consideration of the principles of waves and their interactions.

There is a second important reason to delve deeply into AF: we don't currently have adequate treatments. The inadequacy is in part due to our inability to identify what drives AF in individual patients. There is still wide disagreement among the "experts" as to what the mechanism of AF in humans is.

What type of problem is fibrillation?

For a long time now, academic institutions have been organized around specific disciplines: biology departments, mathematics departments, etc. This binning has been quite useful, helping to focus intellectual pursuits into discrete groups. There are many types of problems. Some – like "At what angle should I tilt my canon to maximize the distance that my cannonballs fly?" – are mono-disciplinic. Answering this question really only requires Newtonian mechanics. It can be solved entirely within the physics department, without need for outside consultation. There are, however, other types of problems that are more complex and do not lend themselves to analytic solutions (i.e. a formula which takes inputs and produces inevitable outputs). For instance, "How does the spread of electrical activity in the heart become disorganized, producing the abnormal heart rhythm, atrial fibrillation?" This is a problem that, as we shall see, simply cannot be solved by plugging numbers into an equation. It isn't that there is an equation out there waiting to be derived but currently too complicated for our not-yet-up-to-the-task brains. Rather, it is that this is an entirely different type of problem, which simply cannot be solved with a formula. That may seem strange. Surely we live in a universe where the laws of physics determine what can and can't happen? This is true; there are rules. Not just *anything* can happen. It turns out that just because there is no formula directly describing how a system evolves does *not* mean that there are no rules governing the system's behavior. It also does not mean that we can't understand how the system works, or that we can't use this understanding to manipulate the system in a predictable way.

There are problems that involve "complex, non-linear, dynamic systems." These types of problems are significantly more slippery when subjected to inquisition. Let's talk about a classic example, the weather. There are laws of physics that constrain what can happen. But alas, the cuffs are not on too tightly: there is an awful lot that can happen. In fact, even if you make a gazillion measurements about the weather *now* (like temperature, wind speed, butterfly wing flappings), you would still be very hard pressed to figure out what the weather will be like *in a week*. And certainly, you'd know almost nothing at all about the weather in a month.

Why is that? Surely weather is simply the result of a bunch of air molecules[1] and water droplets banging into each other? And if that's true, and we know that, say, force equals mass times acceleration, we can simply calculate what happens next, and then next, and then… until we arrive at tomorrow, right? Well, yes and no. We *can* figure out the result of each individual interaction (air molecule vs. air molecule), but there are a bunch of them. So, it is theoretically possible yet completely impractical.

There's a subtle wrinkle in the story. You can't plug a bunch of numbers into a formula and simply use 24 hours instead of one millisecond[2] and derive what the status of things will be at some arbitrary point in the future. You have to put one millisecond into your formula, derive the answer (what the state of things will be next), and then you plug that answer back into your formula and ask about the *next* moment. This is an important distinction. There's no jumping ahead, you have to figure things out *iteratively*. And it gets worse. This process of iterative, stepwise calculation is linear, meaning you do one thing and then another and then another sequentially. These sorts of things are far less complex than systems in which things happen in parallel. We can't simply follow a single air molecule from one moment to the next until some future time, because we need to know what *other* air molecules it will hit, where they will be coming from, and with how much force. And to know that, we need to know what air molecules *those* air molecules were hit by, etc., etc., etc. This is

---

[1] Is air a molecule?
[2] The actual time interval required depends upon the dynamics of the process you are studying.

a non-linear system: what happens to any component of the system *depends upon* what happens to all the other components of the system.[3]

When you think about what our predecessors figured out and handed down in the halls of science, a *lot* more linear problems have been solved than non-linear ones. Why? Because they're easier to solve. But there are ways to address non-linear problems. An interesting aspect of non-linear problems is that, often, small changes in the state of their elements can very quickly result in dramatic changes in outcome. With many elements that are highly sensitive to initial conditions, it can seem that a system is entirely random and therefore not rule-bound. This is captured in the popular expression the "butterfly effect." But "randomness" and "rule-based" are not mutually exclusive notions.

It's pretty hard to figure out what will happen when you flip a coin once, but it's much easier to figure out what will happen if you flip it many, many times. Statistics may be boring, but it is extremely *useful* (and clever). Statistics allows one to wring the most out of what appears to be no information. When it comes to poor data, *more* is actually better!

Structure of the book

Explaining atrial fibrillation is challenging. It's hard to know where to start, because understanding each part of the story seems to depend upon understanding some other part of the story. The issue is that AF is a complex, non-linear process; everything *is* interdependent. The way I've chosen to structure the story is to talk about individual parts: the basic physiology of propagation and reentry ("rules of the game"), followed by the various mechanisms that can drive AF. Next I'll discuss the higher-order dynamics of fibrillation, how the parts interact.

All this information would be for naught if we could not make use of it to treat our patients. To do that, we need to determine what's driving fibrillation in individual patients. So, I'll cover how we can map AF; fibrillation poses some specific challenges for electrode mapping. Finally, it's necessary but not sufficient simply to have a "picture" of fibrillation in our patient. I'll finish with how to leverage our understanding of AF dynamics to intervene and alter atrial physiology to prevent fibrillation.

---

[3] Ahhh, that *is* more complicated.

Acknowledgments

There are several people who have contributed to the work that is described throughout this text. They are the people I refer to when I say that work was done at "our" institution or that "we" did a study. These are we:

Jason Bates and Oliver Bates contributed mightily to the development of the computational model that we use in our lab. Both contributed to the studies we performed with the model as well. All of the following were instrumental in the various studies we've performed, which inform the pages of this book: Bryce Benson, Richard Carrick, Nicole Habel, Nathaniel Thompson, Daniel Correa de Sa, Justin Stinnett-Donnelly, Philip Bileau, Ethan Tischler, Keryn Palmer, Pierre Znojkiewicz, Joachim Müller, Jeffrey Buzas, Arshia Noori, Nicholas Hardin, Steve Bell, James Calame, Vadim Petrov-Kondratov, Bryan Mason, Shruti Sharma, Gagan Mirchandani, Daniel Lustgarten, Deborah Janks, Andreas Karnbach, Susan Calame, Laura Unger, and Srinath Yeshwant. I'd also like to thank Ashley LaScala for her help preparing the manuscript.

My mentor, Burton Sobel, requires special mention for the tremendous role he played in the evolution of both the ideas and the lab group.

PART I
Building blocks of fibrillation

Excitation and propagation

Heart cells have the capacity to be excited or quiescent and while they are excited they cannot be re-excited, i.e. they are refractory. Interestingly, most myocytes will just sit there quiescently unless or until you specifically excite them. Heart cells are generally followers, not leaders. "Command and control" is basically in the sinus node pacemaker cells and everything "works" because there is an orderly spread of the information "hey, beat now" through the remainder of the heart. What's important to know is that the sinus node is not directly wired to each and every myocyte (which would guarantee coordinated excitation/contraction). The situation is actually far more precarious than that. The sinus node cells become excited because they have the capacity to do so, spontaneously. Their neighbors do not have that functionality; they sit quiescent. So, when the sinus cells depolarize, there is a voltage gradient between them and their neighbors. Because the cells are electrically connected (via gap junctions), when there is a voltage gradient, intercellular current flows. *This* current causes membrane depolarization of the neighboring cell(s) and, if it's sufficient to raise the membrane potential to the sodium channel activation threshold, *the neighbor* will become excited. This cell has its own neighbors, and the process repeats such that a wave of successive excitation propagates through the interconnected syncytium of heart muscle cells, *continuing to propagate as long as there are excitable but unexcited neighbors*. "Excitable" means capable of

Understanding Atrial Fibrillation, First Edition. Peter Spector.
© 2020 John Wiley & Sons Ltd. Published 2020 by John Wiley & Sons Ltd.

being excited (something that is not true, for example, with scar or valve tissue); "but unexcited" means that the cell has not already been excited.

Propagation of excitation is very much like the game of dominoes: where propagation leads has a lot to do with how the dominoes are arranged. If we imagine a single line of "dominoes," it's pretty straightforward to see how propagation works. The first cell excites the second, which excites the third, and so on down the line until the last cell is reached. At that point there are no more cells to excite and propagation stops. Things in the heart are more complicated, because the cells aren't connected in single lines, they are arranged in a complex three-dimensional (3D) network. The same rules apply, though: when a cell becomes excited, it excites its excitable but unexcited neighbors. The result is the heart's rhythm.

At this point we have to dig a little deeper into something that we glossed over in the last paragraph. Remember "if that current is sufficient to raise its membrane potential to threshold…"?

Source-sink relationships

It is instructive to think of excited cells as a **source** of current that can be delivered to unexcited cells, which we can think of as a **sink** into which that current is "poured." You can think about this process by picturing buckets (Figure 1A). If the excited cells deliver enough current to raise the sink cells' membrane voltage to threshold, an action potential will result; the sink cell then becomes part of the source for the next cell. If there isn't enough current to depolarize the sink to threshold… no action potential is produced and propagation stops. In the bucket analogy, picture a line of buckets, all connected via tubes (gap junctions) from bottom to bottom (Figure 1B). When current flows (via gap junctions) from source to sink cell 1, some of that current results in depolarization of sink cell 1, but as sink cell 1 depolarizes, a voltage gradient forms between it and *its neighbor* sink cell 2. So, some of the source current flows right through sink cell 1 into sink cell 2. This leaves less current to depolarize sink cell 1. If the sink is larger than the source (e.g. one source cell delivering current to multiple sink cells; Figure 1B), there is "source-sink mismatch" and propagation can fail. Even when there is enough source current to bring the sink cells to threshold, if current is flowing into *multiple* sink cells, the rate of depolarization will be slower. It therefore takes longer to reach threshold and, as a consequence, takes longer before the leading edge of excitation moves forward. So,

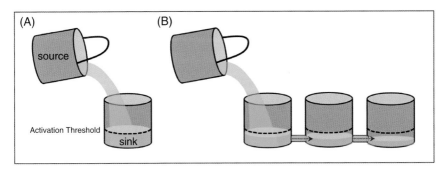

Figure 1 **Source-sink balance**. (A) We can think of excited cells as the *source* of current and unexcited cells as the *sink* into which that current flows. As current flows into the cell, the membrane voltage rises; when it reaches the activation threshold, the cell is excited. (B) Gap junctions connect sink cells, causing progressive dilution of source current; less of the current is available to depolarize the first sink cell due to flow into neighboring sink cells. Depolarization is slower. *Source*: Modified with permission from [1].

reduced source-sink balance decreases conduction velocity; further reduction leads to conduction failure.

What determines source-sink balance?

The determinants of source-sink balance have very important implications for atrial fibrillation (AF). The size of the source is related in part to the number of cells that are excited:[1] two cells deliver more current than one. The size of the sink is related to the number of sink cells:

it's easier for a source cell to depolarize one cell than two. The intercellular resistance influences how far source current passively flows (i.e. how many neighbors' neighbors are divvying up the source current).[2] The *relative number of source and sink cells* can be a function of tissue architecture. At the point where a narrow bundle of cells connects to a much broader sheet of cells (for example where a pectinate muscle inserts into the epicardial layer of cells), there is a sudden increase in sink size (Figure 2); this can be a site of slowed conduction or conduction block [2].

---

[1] Action potential duration also influences source size because the source is not really current, it is actually the total amount of *charge* that is delivered. Longer action potential durations (APDs) provide a larger gradient for a longer time and hence a larger amount of total current.

[2] There are other influences like outward currents that offset the depolarizing effect of intercellular current (for a review, refer to *Understanding Clinical Cardiac Electrophysiology* [1]).

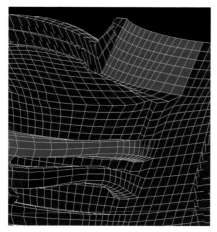

Figure 2 **Tissue architecture and source-sink balance**. Due to source-sink mismatch, conduction slowing or block can occur at the junction where a smaller group of cells meets a larger group, e.g. where pectinate fibers connect to the atrial wall. *Source*: Reproduced with permission from Visible Electrophysiology LLC.

Propagation and reentry

There is nothing special about the connections from the sinus node, through the atrium to the atrioventricular (AV) node, and on through the ventricles. *Any excited cell will excite any excitable and unexcited neighbor.* This is why you can pace the heart from pretty much anywhere you choose. It is also the cause of a lot of trouble. If there happens to be a conduction path that leads in a loop back to where it started, and if the amount of time for the propagating wave to travel around the loop is longer than the refractory period of all the cells in the loop, there is no reason that propagation *will ever end.* This is **reentry:** *perpetual propagation around a closed loop.* When you think about it, it's not surprising that people get arrhythmias; it's amazing that they ever have normal rhythm. But the reason we are not always in some reentrant rhythm is that the conditions for reentry aren't often met.

Requirements for reentry

Because cells have a finite refractory period following excitation, a wave cannot reverse direction and double back over the path it has just traveled. This would require (at the turnaround point) that an excited cell reexcite the very neighbor that excited it. But *that* cell is refractory because it was just excited. Instead, for reentry to occur, there must be two distinct paths that travel away from and back toward any given point. There must be uninterrupted connections along this entire path, i.e. it must be a closed loop or, in electrophysiology (EP) parlance, a **circuit**. But a circuit alone is not sufficient to produce reentry. If a wave of excitation travels down *both* paths of the circuit, the waves will reach each other on the far side of the circuit, collide, and be annihilated (Figure 3A). Waves can't propagate through each other for the same reason they can't reverse direction: cells at the leading edge of excitation are refractory. Reentry requires not simply a circuit, but also conduction that travels down only one path and not the other – a **unidirectional conduction block** (Figure 3B). There is one final requirement for reentry: the wave length must be less than the path length around the circuit (**wave length < path length**, or WL < PL). The "wave length" is the physical distance from the leading edge of excitation to the trailing edge of recovery. If the wave length is longer than the path length, the wave front will arrive where it started, before the cells there have recovered from refractoriness. When this happens, there are no

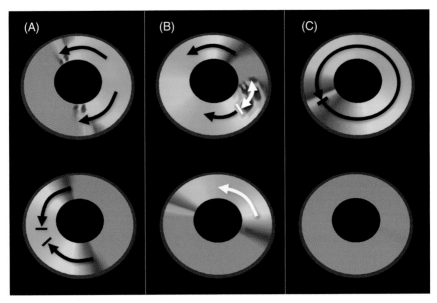

Figure 3 A circuit is not the only requirement for reentry. (A) A paced wave (black arrows) conducts both clockwise and counter-clockwise around the circuit. With bidirectional conduction, waves will meet, collide, and be annihilated on the far side of a circuit. (B) A premature paced beat S2 (white arrow) is delivered shortly after the initial paced beat S1 (black arrows). S2 is delivered *closer to the tail of the clockwise wave*, and thus blocks in the clockwise but not counter-clockwise direction. Following unidirectional block, reentry is possible. (C) If wave length is greater than path length, the wave will collide with its own tail and annihilate itself. *Source*: Reproduced with permission from Visible Electrophysiology LLC.

more "excitable but unexcited" cells, and propagation ceases (Figure 3C).

What makes a circuit?

Anything that results in two separate paths that are connected at both ends makes a circuit. The simplest to conceive are physical circuits like atrial flutter, where the "paths" are the tissue surrounding the tricuspid annulus and the thing that separates the paths is the valve itself. Also pretty straightforward is the circuit in orthodromic reentry: atrium, atrioventricular node (AVN)/His-Purkinje system (HPS), ventricle, accessory pathway (AP), and back to the atrium. Here the thing that "separates" the paths… is all the things that separate those paths: the AV annuli separating atrium (A) from ventricle (V) electrically, etc. These are two examples of **structural reentrant circuits**. There can also be **functional reentrant circuits**. In these, functional conduction failure separates cells from each other, creating the "paths." In a functional circuit, conduction fails not because of a structure that has permanently unexcitable cells (e.g. valve rings or scar tissue), but rather due to some "functional" reason (e.g. they are refractory from having recently been excited).

Source-sink balance and rotors

Tissue architecture is not the only thing that can influence the number of source cells versus sink cells. Wave *shape* has an impact on source-sink balance. A planar wave has a 1 : 1 ratio of source cells to sink cells (Figure 4A), while a curved wave has more sink cells than source cells (Figure 4B). This means that *as wave curvature increases, conduction velocity decreases*. It also means that at a certain point curvature is steep enough that source-sink mismatch leads to conduction failure. This is the physiology that underlies rotors (Figure 4C).

Imagine a premature beat arising in the middle of an expanse of tissue, colliding with the tail of a wave propagating across the tissue (Figure 5A). The wave breaks, because one portion encounters refractory tissue at the prior wave's tail; we now have two wave ends in the middle of the tissue (Figure 5B).[3] For cells in the center of this wave, there is a 1 : 1 source-sink balance (each cell provides current to the cell immediately in front of it). But as we get to the ends of the wave, the cell at the wave tip provides current to the cell in front *and* to the side

---

[3] If the two broken wave ends are close enough to each other, they can fuse back into one wave.

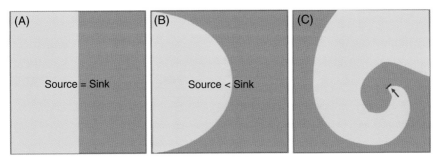

Figure 4 **Curvature and source-sink balance.** (A) In a planar wave (yellow), source = sink. (B) With a curved wave, source < sink. (C) At the point of maximum curvature (arrow), source-sink mismatch causes block, around which rotation occurs. *Source*: Reproduced with permission from Visible Electrophysiology LLC.

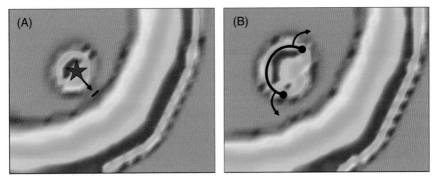

Figure 5 **Wave break causes rotor formation**. (A) A premature atrial contraction (star) behind a receding wave front causes wave break where wave front meets wave tail (arrow). (B) Two "free" wave ends are formed adjacent to the site of wave break, leading to counter-rotating rotors. *Source*: Reproduced with permission from Visible Electrophysiology LLC.

(Figure 5B). The end of the wave front will therefore propagate more slowly than the middle (it will take longer for the wave tip to excite its neighbors). This creates a curved wave front. As the wave front curves, the "inside" of the curve (nearest the tip) will propagate more slowly, so the curvature will increase. This will continue to a point at which the curve is steep enough that the wave tip cannot excite the innermost cells (due to source-sink mismatch). The unexcited cells at the center form an obstacle[4]

---

[4] A functional obstacle.

around which rotation occurs;[5] the functional reentrant circuit that results is called a **rotor**.[6] Think of running through the woods and tripping on a branch. Your feet are suddenly "propagating" slower than your head and you "rotate" around the branch.[7]

Wave length

Wave length is a critical concept in AF, so we'll take a moment to go over it here. Wave length is literally a length: it is the physical distance from the leading edge of excitation (the wave front) to the trailing edge of repolarization (wave tail). Wave length (mm) is simply the product of the **velocity** (mm/ms) and the APD (ms).

$$WL = CV * APD$$

The wave front travels at a certain rate (the conduction velocity, CV) and how far it gets in the amount of time it takes the first cell to repolarize (the APD) is the wave *length*. If the APD is longer, there is more time for the wave front to travel before the tail repolarizes (longer wave length). If the conduction velocity is faster, the wave front can travel farther during the time it takes for the tail to repolarize (Figure 6), thus increased conduction velocity also increases wave length.

Wave length is influenced by cell and tissue properties *as well as* by wave shape.

Tissue Properties: Interstitial fibrosis, gap junctions, fiber orientation,[8] and inward current densities all

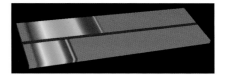

Figure 6 **Wave length and conduction velocity**. The tissue on the top and that on the bottom have the same action potential durations (APD), but the top has faster conduction velocity. The wave *front* has gotten farther (top) because it conducts more rapidly. The wave *tails* are at the same location, because they are repolarizing *at the same rate* (APD is the same top and bottom). Therefore the wave *length* is longer on the top. *Source*: Reproduced with permission from Visible Electrophysiology LLC.

---

[5] Because there are two waves (one on either side of the break), there will be two counter-rotating rotors. As we will see later, if the wave tips are too close together, there will be source-sink mismatch as propagation tries to emerge from between the cores. Conduction fails, and both rotors annihilate.

[6] Rotor terminology is somewhat loose: some studies will refer to the center of reentry as a rotor, and the "arms" that emanate outward from the center as spiral waves. Others use the terms interchangeably.

[7] There won't be reentry because the ground will interrupt the "circuit."

---

[8] Fiber orientation influences conduction velocity *because* gap junctions are not evenly distributed along the cell: there are more junctions at the ends than along the sides of cells.

influence conduction velocity; the balance of inward and outward currents influences APD. Some of the outward currents are intrinsic transmembrane currents (via ion channels) and some are "electrotonic" currents, leaving the cell via gap junctions.[9]

Wave Shape: Due to its effect on electrotonic currents, wave shape[10] also influences conduction velocity and APD.

The source-sink balance along a wave is influenced by the *curvature* of the wave. With high curvature, sink is larger than source (e.g. toward the center of a rotor), so there are greater outward (electrotonic) currents and therefore the action potential is shorter than that same cell's APD would have been if it were "contained" in a planar wave (Figure 7) [3].

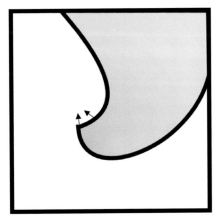

Figure 7 Electrotonic currents, wave length, and conduction velocity. Wave length is shorter at the tip of the rotor because more electrotonic current (arrows) is spreading from the excited cells to the unexcited sink (expediting repolarization).

Wave length, path length, and reentry

One of the "requirements of reentry" is that wave length must be less than or equal to path length. But the *impact* of wave length versus path length on reentry differs between structural and functional circuits. In a structural circuit, if the whole wave front meets the whole wave tail at the same time (Figure 8A), there will be no excitable cells and reentry will terminate. Consider what happens when the wave length at the center of a rotor is longer than the path length around the rotor core (Figure 8B). In this case the circuit itself is not fixed

---

[9] We can distinguish the *intrinsic* APD from the *actual* APD. "Intrinsic" is the APD that a cell would have in the absence of the influence of its neighbors (i.e. due to transmembrane currents but not electrotonic currents). The "actual" APD includes the effects of intercellular currents.

[10] The shape of a wave is not an intrinsic property of the tissue, it is determined by how the tissue happens to be excited. For example, a concentric wave (e.g. emanating from a focal pacing site) vs. the V-shaped wave front where two concentric waves collide and fuse.

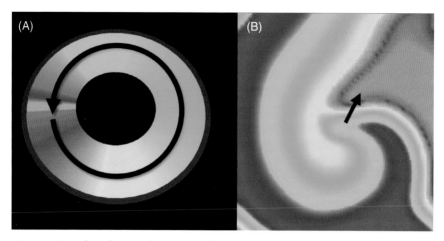

Figure 8 Wave length vs. path length. (A) In a structural circuit, if wave length is greater than path length, the entire wave front meets the entire wave tail and reentry terminates. (B) In a functional circuit the wave front and wave tail are not parallel; note the shape of the excitable gap (gray). Thus, if wave length is longer than path length in a functional circuit, the wave *tip* meets its own wave tail, then travels along the recovering tail until sufficient recovery allows rotation; the core meanders. *Source*: Reproduced with permission from [1].

in space by anatomic features (as is the case in a structural circuit), *and* the wave front and wave tail are not parallel, so only a portion of the wave's front meets the refractory cells of the wave's tail. The wave *tip* meets its tail and propagates along the tail, exciting recovered cells immediately behind the wave tail. As the tip moves along the wave tail, the tail itself is moving away from the wave front (as cells repolarize) and eventually the wave tip can rotate again. Depending upon the path of the moving wave tip, the rotor can remain stable or meander through the tissue.

Restitution

APD is not a fixed value, it varies depending upon rate of excitation; the faster a cell is excited, the shorter its APD. Indirectly, this is the reason that the QT interval has to be corrected for heart rate. The details of restitution are not critical to our story, but the impact of the *slope* of restitution is important. The restitution curve plots APD against prior diastolic interval (Figure 9). If the slope of the line relating these two is greater than 1, APD changes a lot, even when the diastolic interval

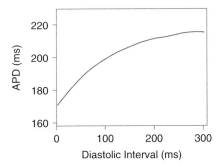

Figure 9 Restitution curve. Action potential duration (APD; y-axis) decreases as diastolic interval (x-axis) decreases. *Source*: Reproduced with permission from [1].

changes a little. There is a direct relationship between diastolic interval and APD (Figure 9). When the slope of the restitution curve is steep, small changes in diastolic interval cause large changes in APD. Because of the reciprocal relationship between diastolic interval and APD (diastolic interval plus APD equals cycle length), oscillation can develop over sequential beats. APD shortening causes diastolic interval lengthening, which causes APD lengthening, etc. When the slope of the restitution curve is greater than 1, these oscillations can amplify and cause wave break (secondary to refractoriness). This can be an important factor in fibrillation. In fact, it has been demonstrated that flattening the restitution slope (<1) with bretylium can prevent wave break and fibrillation, and even

convert ventricular fibrillation to ventricular tachycardia (Figure 10) [4–6]. Monophasic action potential recordings have been used to measure APD in patients with paroxysmal and persistent AF. In paroxysmal AF patients, restitution slope was greater than 1 near the pulmonary veins and facilitated initiation of AF by single premature atrial contractions (PACs). In patients with persistent AF, there was rate-dependent variability of conduction near the veins which flattened the restitution curve and PACs failed to initiate fibrillation [7].[11]

Initiating reentry

Now that we've gone over many of the building blocks of reentry, let's discuss how reentry starts in the first place. The easiest case to consider is structural reentry. The mere presence of a circuit does not necessitate reentry *around the circuit*. Think of a patient with an accessory pathway. In sinus rhythm, a wave propagates

---

[11] Michael Franz has postulated that the normal *ventricular* restitution is actually triphasic (a steep initial slope, transient decline, and then slow increase in APD). He proposes that the initial steep slope of the curve (at the shortest diastolic intervals) promotes more rapid shifting of the APD to the flatter portion of the curve, stabilizing oscillations. Thus, flattening can paradoxically prolong alternans (alternating long and short APD) [8].

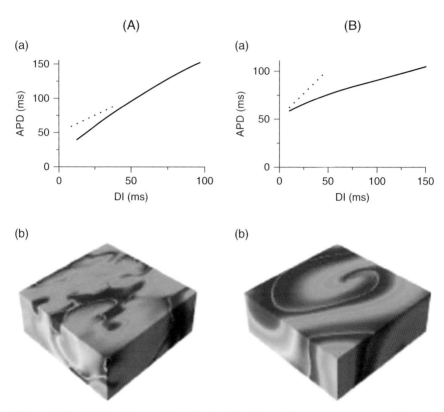

Figure 10 Restitution slope and fibrillation. The slope of the restitution curve influences the stability of waves. When the restitution slope is >1, oscillations in the refractory period tend to amplify until wave break occurs. A (left column): (a) steep restitution curve; (b) complex rotors with multiple wave breaks. B (right column): (a) flatter restitution curve; (b) more organized rotors without wave break along the spiral arms. *Source*: Modified from [4].

through the atria to the AVN *and* to the AP. Both will generate waves of depolarization in the ventricles, which will collide somewhere in the ventricle and annihilate each other; there won't be reentry (Figure 11A). Reentry requires that propagation use either the AVN/HPS or the AP but not both (i.e. there must be unidirectional block). If a premature beat arises near the AP *before* the AP has recovered from the refractoriness of the prior beat, the PAC will block at, rather than conduct through, the AP (Figures 11B and C). If the PAC wave takes sufficiently long to reach the AVN, such that the node has recovered from refractoriness, it will

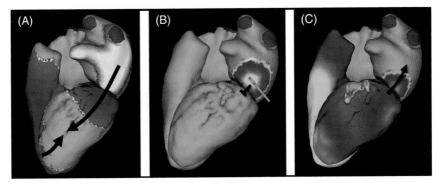

Figure 11 Unidirectional block initiates reentry. (A) Sinus beat – antegrade waves from the left free wall accessory pathway (AP) and the His-Purkinje system (HPS) collide, hence no reentry (left bundle branch block is shown to accentuate pre-excitation). (B) A premature paced beat, from near the AP site, blocks at the AP, but (C) conducts via the HPS. It then conducts retrograde via the AP, initiating reentry. *Source*: Reproduced with permission from Visible Electrophysiology LLC.

conduct to the HPS. This is an example of unidirectional block. It can occur due to waves arriving at two paths *with different refractory periods* at the same time,[12] or due to waves arriving at two paths with the same refractory period *at different times* (e.g. by pacing closer to the AP than the AVN).

Let's return to our patient with a blocked PAC and an AP. We now have a wave traveling down the AVN but not the AP. When that wave reaches the ventricular side of the AP, it will have recovered from refractoriness (the ventricular side was excited by the sinus beat *before* the PAC).[13] If, by the time the retrograde wave traverses the AP, the atrial tissue adjacent to the AP has recovered from the PAC, it can reenter the atrium.

We've already discussed how functional reentry can be initiated: wave break. In this case the *wave break creates unidirectional conduction* – propagation in the direction of rotation and not in the opposite direction – *and creates the circuit itself* – the unexcited cells at the core (source-sink mismatch) separate the cells surrounding the core, producing the circuit (Figure 12) [9].

---

[12] If a wave arrives simultaneously at two paths, with the same refractory period (i.e. the same APD) but which were previously excited at different times, block can occur in one (the more recently excited) and conduct in the other.

---

[13] Because the AP was blocked, the ventricular side didn't get activated by the PAC, it was activated by the sinus beat that preceded the PAC.

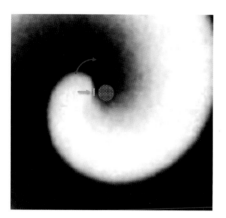

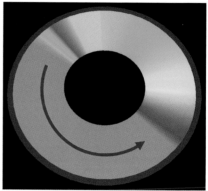

Figure 12 **Wave break creates unidirectional block *and* a circuit**. Tight curvature at the wave tip causes conduction block (green arrow) due to source-sink mismatch. This produces an unexcited core (red circle) around which rotation propagates (red arrow). *Source*: Modified from [9].

Figure 13 **Circuit topology**. A circuit is a spatial relationship that places the leading edge of a wave in electrical continuity with the trailing edge. As a result, the leading edge of excitation has a continuous supply of excitable cells. *Source*: Reproduced with permission from Visible Electrophysiology LLC.

Getting back to basics, reentry is continuous propagation, and continuous propagation requires the leading edge of excitation to continually encounter excitable cells. This, ultimately, is what the "reentry requirements" insure: a circuit, unidirectional block, and WL < PL all *permit the wave front ongoing access to excitable cells*.

A Deeper look at circuits

A circuit is fundamentally a spatial relationship between excitable and excited cells, such that *the leading edge of excitation is in continuity with the trailing edge where cells recover excitability* (Figure 13).[14] The wave front is constantly consuming excitable cells; in order for reentry to be perpetuated, cells must constantly regain excitability *in front of the leading edge of propagation*. What's the big deal? Cells always regain excitability, they depolarize, and at the end of the action potential, they repolarize and are excitable again. What is special (or particular) about a circuit is the spatial conformation, which places the reexcitable cells *in the path of the excitation wave* (Figure 13).

---

[14] "Continuity" in the sense of unobstructed access to; not to be confused with wave front *touches* wave tail (i.e. WL = PL).

Wave ends, boundaries, and circuits
Imagine a planar wave front on a flat sheet of cells (Figure 14A). The wave front has two ends, and each end is "on" a boundary. If you trace the boundary forward from one end, you will come to the other end without leaving the boundary; both ends *are on the same boundary*. In this configuration there is no continuity between the cells in front of the wave and those behind it. The cells in front will

be "consumed" (by excitation), the cells behind the wave will recover excitability, but the wave front has no access to them. Propagation will cease as soon as the excitable cells in front of the wave are used up. Now, imagine a sheet of tissue with a hole in its center (Figure 14B and C). A wave front traveling around the hole will have one wave end on the outer boundary (edge of the tissue) and the other wave end on the inner boundary.

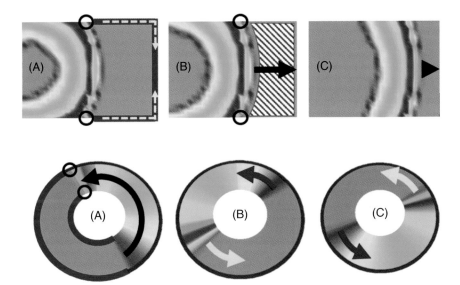

Figure 14 **Topology wave ends and boundaries.** Top: (A) When both wave ends (black circles) are on the same boundary, the region of excitable cells (B) – the red and white striped region – will be consumed. (C) The new supply of excitable cells, due to recovery *behind* the wave tail, is not accessible to the wave front, so propagation is extinguished. Reentry is not possible. Bottom: (A) When wave ends are on different boundaries (black circles), the wave front has direct access to perpetually renewed excitable cells. (B) At the wave front, cells are consumed (yellow arrow) at the same rate as they recover at the wave tail (blue arrow). Propagation can continue indefinitely. (C) Because excitation and recovery occur at the same rate, the distance between wave front and wave tail remains fixed. *Source*: Modified from [1].

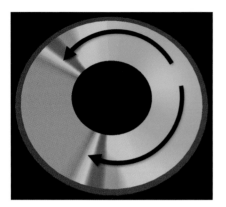

Figure 15 Reentry requires unidirectional block. When waves travel along both sides of a circuit (arrows), they will collide and annihilate each other, precluding reentry. *Source*: Reproduced with permission from Visible Electrophysiology LLC.

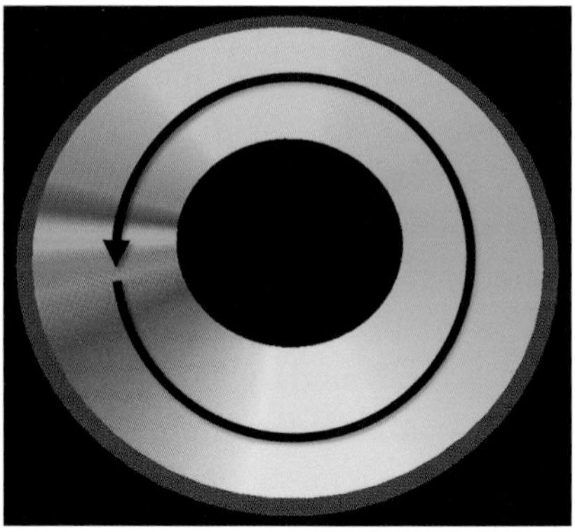

Figure 16 Reentry requires that wave length is less than path length, otherwise head meets tail and reentry terminates. *Source*: Reproduced with permission from Visible Electrophysiology LLC.

The fact that the two wave ends *are on different boundaries* places the recovering cells in the path of the wave front.

Actually, I pulled a fast one there. The fact that the wave ends are on different boundaries is necessary, but not sufficient for reentry. If there is *another wave* propagating along the opposite side of the hole (Figure 15), then there *is not an uninterrupted path between wave front and wave tail*.[15] The two waves will eventually and *inevitably* collide and propagation will cease. Rather than saying reentry requires unidirectional block, it is perhaps more accurate to say it

requires *unidirectional conduction*.[16] A circuit *is* a continuous connection between excited cells and recovering cells; a physical "circuit" alone doesn't necessarily meet this criterion, as there must also be a functional connection.

If we consider the final reentry requirement, WL<PL, this is effectively just the "functional connection" story again. Only in this case, a wave's own tail provides functional block to the wave front, so that it is *not* in continuity with recovering cells (Figure 16). A circuit is two physically connected *conduction* paths.

---

[15] For either wave.

[16] Unidirectional block is one way to achieve unidirectional conduction. Unidirectional conduction is the "real" requirement.

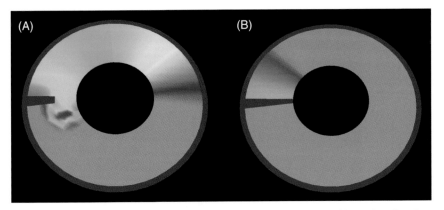

Figure 17 **Termination requires complete circuit transection**. (A) An ablation line that does not completely transect the circuit leaves a path for propagation, allowing continued reentry. If there is a narrow gap through the ablation line, slow propagation can decrease wave length and stabilize reentry. (B) With complete transection there is no longer a circuit and reentry cannot be supported. *Source*: Reproduced with permission from Visible Electrophysiology LLC.

Terminating reentry

Once started, how does reentry ever terminate? The preceding discussion provides the answer(s). Anything that *interrupts* the circuit will terminate reentry. Termination can be achieved through **physical** disruption of the paths, i.e. ablation, which places permanently non-conducting tissue across the circuit. "Across" must be *all the way* across: an ablation line that is only partway across the circuit leaves an intact connection (Figure 17) and propagation can sneak by.[17]

Circuit interruption can be **functional** (and hence transient[18]). This is how anti-arrhythmic drugs work. Class III drugs prolong the refractory period; if they prolong it sufficiently, the wave length will exceed the path length and head meets tail, causing circuit interruption and termination. Adenosine (or vagal maneuvers) cause functional block in the AVN, another version of functional circuit interruption. Sodium channel blockade can decrease excitability sufficiently to cause conduction failure.

A fortuitously timed premature wave reaching the circuit will split

---

[17] In fact, partial ablation often creates a zone of source-sink mismatch which slows conduction, decreasing wave length and making termination *less* likely. Slowed conduction is why "wounding," but not destroying, an accessory pathway can result in incessant orthodromic reciprocating tachycardia.

[18] Functional circuit interruption does not preclude reentry in the future (it simply terminates *an episode*), whereas ablation eliminates the structural circuit permanently.

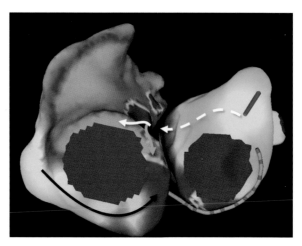

Figure 18 Circuit penetration by a paced wave. A paced wave (dashed white arrow) enters the circuit of typical atrial flutter (black arrow), where it splits into an orthodromic wave (solid white arrow) and an antidromic wave (green arrow). The clockwise paced wave (green arrow) and the counter-clockwise flutter wave (black arrow) will collide and annihilate each other, while the counter-clockwise paced wave (white arrow) will continue around the circuit *before* the flutter wave otherwise would have. *Source*: Reproduced with permission from Visible Electrophysiology LLC.

and propagate *both* ways: one wave in the direction of the reentry wave ("orthodromic" wave) and one in the opposite direction ("antidromic" wave). The antidromic wave *must* collide with the oncoming orthodromic reentry wave (Figure 18); these two will annihilate each other. If the orthodromic wave arrives at just the right time (relative to the reentry wave) it will collide with the tail of the reentry wave, in which case all waves have been annihilated: antidromic premature annihilates itself (i) *and* the orthodromic reentry wave (ii), while the orthodromic premature wave annihilates itself (iii) against the tail of the orthodromic reentry wave. If the orthodromic premature wave does not collide with the tail of the receding reentry wave, there will be nothing to prevent it from propagating.[19] At first glance it appears that reentry has not been terminated, but in reality it has, it's just that it was immediately reinitiated by the orthodromic portion of the same wave that terminated it. This is called resetting (because the reentry has been "reset" by the premature wave, such that

---

[19] This happens if it arrives a little later, such that the reentry wave's tail has already passed by.

activation occurs sooner than it otherwise would have[20]).

There is yet one more response to an external wave colliding with a structural reentrant wave. If the incoming wave's front collides only with the innermost portion of the reentry wave's tail, the entire wave front does not collide with the entire wave tail. Then, much like a functional rotor (with $WL > PL$), the wave tip will travel along the receding wave tail and "lift off" the central obstacle of the structural reentrant circuit. If the wave tip is able to turn before it reaches the edge of the tissue (as the wave tail recedes), then the structural reentrant circuit will have been converted into a functional circuit [10].

---

[20] If you work it through, the premature wave reached the beginning of the circuit *before* the original reentry wave and hence started around the circuit sooner than it would have; the tachycardia is *advanced*.

PART II
Atrial fibrillation mechanisms

The evolution of current concepts

The following is a brief synopsis of how we arrived at our current "understanding" of atrial fibrillation (AF) mechanisms. It is not intended to be an exhaustive review of the literature, but rather a narrative that touches on the milestones, putting into context contemporary controversies.

The study of fibrillation began before the recording of electrocardiograms (EKGs) – and well before intracardiac electrical recordings. Despite the rudimentary access to data, theories about the mechanism of fibrillation were remarkably insightful. In 1887, physiologist John McWilliam performed a series of studies of fibrillation in "the hearts of the dog, cat, rabbit, rat, mouse, hedgehog and fowl."[1] The studies were based solely upon visual inspection of contraction in hearts exposed to "faradic"[2] stimulation. He drew a very important conclusion that relates to fibrillation as a complex dynamic non-linear phenomenon: "The arrhythmic fibrillar contraction is *not dependent* on the destruction or paralysis of a *co-ordinating centre*" (emphasis added) [11]. However, almost from the beginning there has been debate as to the mechanism(s) of fibrillation. The name wasn't even settled upon for a long time. Neither, for that matter, was the understanding

---

[1] It is a miracle that he was able to learn *anything*, given all the time he must have spent interacting with the IACUC.
[2] Low-intensity and low-frequency alternating current.

---

that the phenomenon observed in animal hearts had any relation to a human arrhythmia. The name itself, "fibrillation", has its origins in one of the early mechanistic formulations. It was believed that fibrillation (whether atrial or ventricular) was due to multiple ectopic foci. The notion that individual *fibers* could contract independently led to the name *fibrillation* [12].

Cardiologist Sir James Mackenzie used a new method to study fibrillation: recording of the jugular pressure tracing as a surrogate for direct measurement of atrial and ventricular pressure (Figure 19) [13]. He noted that during fibrillation, there was no

wave indicative of atrial contraction; from this he initially concluded that AF was due to atrial paralysis. Subsequently, having observed abrupt restoration of atrial waves (with conversion), he felt that paralysis was unlikely. He postulated that the atrial contraction wave was superimposed upon the larger, ventricular contraction wave and therefore hidden. This, he guessed, was due to the contraction of both arising from between the two, at the AV junction; this is the origin of the term "nodal rhythm." The nodal rhythm hypothesis was widely accepted. Physician Thomas Lewis saw a patient who was in (an actual) nodal rhythm and noted that it was completely regular, while fibrillation is irregular. He concluded that the two were different rhythms. He then employed the string galvanometer (an early EKG) and recognized the irregular F waves during AF that replaced the organized P waves of sinus rhythm. He noted that the QRS complex was similar during sinus and fibrillation and postulated that this meant the rhythm was arising in the atria (Figure 20). He actually placed both electrodes of the galvanometer on the same arm of a patient and determined that the fibrillation waves were not due to a tremor of the arm. He next placed the electrodes directly on the surface of the fibrillating canine atria, finally

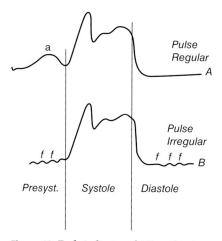

Figure 19 Early indicator of AF mechanism. Recordings of the jugular venous pressure tracing reveals (top) atrial contraction ("a" waves during sinus rhythm) and (bottom) tiny "F" waves (during fibrillation). *Source*: Reproduced with permission from [14].

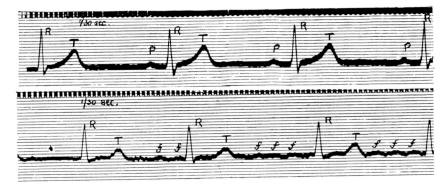

Figure 20 Early electrocardiograms performed by Thomas Lewis. Sinus rhythm (top) and atrial fibrillation (bottom). *Source*: Reproduced with permission from [14].

identifying that the chaotic electrical activity *is* from the atria. Pleased with this explanation, and jumping somewhat prematurely to the conclusion that all was now resolved, he stated: "the proof as I have given it … explains almost all the phenomena which are associated with it as a mechanism" [14].

In the early part of the twentieth century the notion of reentry was first conceived. Initial studies demonstrated reentry in a physically (surgically) created ring of tissue (Figure 21) [15]. Physiologist George Mines noted, even in these early studies, that "On increasing the frequency of excitation, the wave becomes both slower and shorter. Under these circumstances it becomes possible for the whole wave to be present at one time on the muscle column" [15]. He extrapolated his findings to unperturbed cardiac tissue, noting that the syncytial nature of cardiac fibers

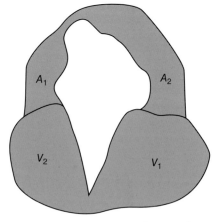

Figure 21 Surgically created circuit. In an early demonstration of reentry, Mines created a circuit for reentry in a tortoise heart. *Source*: Reproduced with permission from [15].

allows for any number of circuits. He also introduced the notion of circuits and unidirectional conduction, "Supposing an excitation to be started in such a closed circuit and supposing for some reason it travels in one direction but not the other" [15]. Finally, he extrapolated the notion of reentry further, intuiting that it was a possible cause of fibrillation [15].

Focal or disseminated?

Lewis's ideas about fibrillation continued to develop and by 1921 he felt that it was the result of a single reentrant driver that could be terminated via use of quinidine: "in auricular fibrillation a circus movement exists in the auricle; that a single wave is propagated and revolves perpetually upon a re-entrant path." He went on to say that the effect of quinidine "is a lengthening of the refractory period … thus rendering the gap between the crest and the wake of the circulating wave shorter and eventually abolishing it altogether" [16]. So that you don't think that controversy and discord are solely a modern phenomenon, Mackenzie had this to say: "The mere fact that in auricular fibrillation there is a short refractory period does not justify the assumption that the shortened refractory period is the cause of the auricular fibrillation. Trying to stop fibrillation by attempting to lengthen the refractory period is manifestly a procedure which is bound to fail, and is due to a misconception of the nature of the condition."[3]

It was noted by some researchers that fibrillatory contraction could be initiated by electrical stimulation from a fixed site. It was felt that fibrillation was not simply *initiated* from a single site, but also *perpetuated* from this same site. This was tested and demonstrated to not necessarily be true. Physiologist Walter Garrey [17] performed a simple experiment: he initiated fibrillation in a sheet of tissue, then, using scissors, removed the corner from which fibrillation had been initiated. He demonstrated that fibrillation persisted in the absence of its site of initiation. This introduced the important concept that the **initiation and perpetuation mechanisms** for fibrillation *need not* be one and the same.

Having seized upon an effective research tool, a pair of scissors, Garrey proceeded to remove thin strips of tissue from the fibrillating atrial preparation. The strips, once excised, immediately ceased spontaneous electrical activity, but retained the capacity to be stimulated. This indicated that (at least in these studies) *fibrillating muscle fibers were not independent.*[4] He continued in what was perhaps one of the most productive (and least complicated) set of experiments in fibrillation ever conducted. He noted that the

---

[3] Note to self: think twice and publish once.

[4] Otherwise the removed strips would continue to fibrillate.

size of the strips mattered. Sufficiently large strips could continue fibrillating, while smaller ones could not. He (thought to look and) demonstrated that it was not simply the area of the tissue that was the limiting parameter for fibrillation, but also the width. From these observations he concluded (i) that fibrillation was *a reentrant rhythm* (comprising complete circuits of excitation), and (ii) that these circuits *required* a *minimum "turning radius"* and thus could not be sustained in narrow tissue. He also set the stage for the "probabilistic formulation" of fibrillation when he noted that not only was the absolute capacity to support fibrillation dependent upon tissue size/shape, but *the duration of episodes was proportional to tissue mass* [17].

Finally, based upon the observation that the atria (or ventricles) could fibrillate without the opposite chambers fibrillating, Garrey tested the notion that it was simply the width of the His bundle that precluded transmission of fibrillation from one chamber to the other. He took a sheet of fibrillating tissue and made incisions inward from opposite sides of the tissue, then demonstrated that the ability for fibrillation to be transmitted from one side of the connecting channel to the other depended upon the width of the channel (Figure 22).

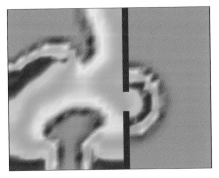

Figure 22 Transmission of fibrillation. A recapitulation of Garrey's "narrow channel can't transmit fibrillation" experiment. The left side of the tissue is fibrillating. The tissue is partially transected (gray lines) and fibrillation does not cross through the narrow channel. Rather, there is focal activation of the right side of the tissue via the left–right connection. *Source*: Reproduced with permission from Visible Electrophysiology LLC.

He noted that the existence of transient and shifting functional block provided the conditions for "a series of ring-like circuits of shifting locations and multiply [sic] complexity" [17]. Just in case you are not yet duly impressed with this paper, he also postulated that unidirectional block (required for initiation of reentry around a ring of turtle ventricular muscle) could result from irregularities in the width of the ring. This presaged the discovery that changes in fiber thickness (among other things) could produce unidirectional conduction block due to source-sink mismatch.

Multiwavelet reentry moves to the forefront

In 1959, Gordon Moe and Junior Abildskov performed a series of experiments in open-chested dogs [18].[5] Their studies underscore several important aspects of the atrial fibrillation story and merit discussion here. In the introduction to the paper, they make a point that I believe is critical and yet still often misinterpreted to this day: **"Since both circus movement and ectopic focus mechanisms have been produced experimentally, it is unrealistic to propose that only one of these mechanisms can exist in patients."** They next made the point that the term atrial fibrillation is applied to "tachycardias so rapid that uniform atrial excitation does not occur" [18]. This implies the important notion that in the discussion of AF mechanisms one must consider that fibrillation need not have a single mechanism; rather, *anything* that causes non-"uniform atrial excitation" is by definition fibrillation. They noted that the irregular activity itself makes it difficult to identify the mechanism of AF. While multiple ectopic foci or a single reentrant driver could clearly drive AF, it seemed unlikely to them that these could last consistently enough to explain long-standing AF [18].

In the canine heart, Moe and Abildskov stimulated the right atrial appendage (RAA) and demonstrated that the response of the atria depended upon the rate of stimulation. Stimulation at "6 or 7" beats per second was uniformly conducted throughout the atria, and when stimulation stopped, excitation immediately stopped. When pacing at "9 to 11" beats per second, activation became "grossly irregular"[6]; and when this occurred, activation often persisted following cessation of pacing. They next performed atrial pacing while simultaneously stimulating the vagal nerves. The result was that AF persisted after cessation of pacing and until several seconds after vagal stimulation was discontinued. They recapitulated Garrey's protocol by clamping off the RAA after fibrillation had been initiated. They found that, so long as there was ongoing vagal stimulation, fibrillation persisted in the absence of electrical continuity between the appendage (where fibrillation had been initiated) and the remainder of the atria [18].

---

[5] Interestingly, I met Junior Abildskov when I applied for my cardiology fellowship at the University of Utah. He told me that he didn't believe I was really interested in research. I was accepted anyway. I've continued to fake an interest for the past 25 years.

[6] I.e. fibrillatory conduction.

Their interpretation of these data was that the *mechanism of fibrillation depends upon experimental conditions*. In the absence of vagal stimulation, AF was focally driven (in this case, pacing); cessation of pacing (or clamping of the appendage) immediately terminated fibrillation. In the presence of vagal stimulation, fibrillation was no longer dependent upon focal firing. Moe and Abildskov expressed doubt that the "self-sustaining" fibrillation could be due to ectopic firing, initiated by the atrial pacing, but located remote from the pacing site. Based upon this "exclusion" of ectopic firing, they felt that vagally mediated AF (in this model) was most consistent with Garrey's "multiple wave hypothesis."

They postulated that vagal stimulation decreases the refractory period of some, but not all, atrial cells. This, they felt, explained the observation that the fastest 1 : 1 conduction rate was the same in the presence or absence of vagal stimulation; since vagal stimulation shortened the refractory period of some but not all cells, the breakdown of 1 : 1 conduction should depend upon the *longest* refractory period (not the shortest). Thus, they expected that the rate threshold for degeneration to fibrillatory conduction would be the same with and without vagal stimulation.

Moe and Abildskov proposed that the average refractory period of atrial cells is reduced by vagal stimulation and that this is why AF perpetuates for longer during vagal stimulation. With shorter waves, more waves can fit on the tissue and the probability of spontaneous termination is decreased (so duration is increased). They pointed out that AF duration will vary directly with (i) atrial mass and (ii) mean conduction velocity, and (iii) inversely with mean refractory period.

They concluded this milestone paper by stating that their data "emphasize the necessity of a definition of fibrillation in terms of mechanism rather than in terms of the gross and superficial criterion of irregularity of electrical events in the atria." They considered that fibrillation could result from focal drivers, ectopic foci, or multi-wavelet reentry, and that "It is conceivable that all possible mechanisms are encountered in the clinic."

While these data were consistent with multi-wavelet reentry[7] as a mechanism of atrial fibrillation, Moe and Abildskov did not prove it. Without the capacity to map atrial activation with any significant sample

---

[7] In this text I use the term "multi-wavelet reentry" interchangeably with the more often used "multiple wave reentry."

density (in 1960), they felt that they could not directly demonstrate multi-wavelet reentry. They therefore sought to create multi-wavelet reentry in a computer model so as to demonstrate that it is a *possible* driver of fibrillation.

In what was to be another landmark paper, they created a "cellular automaton" model, which basically means that they modeled "cells" with rules that capture the behavior of excitable myocytes [19]. They didn't create a model of individual ion channels and combine these within a model of a cell, to elicit the emergent behavior of cardiac action potentials. Instead, they directly modeled cell excitation. A "cell" was actually a representation of a region of cells (not an individual myocyte). These cells had different "states"; they could be excited or quiescent. Once excited, they were refractory to reexcitation for an "absolute refractory period" and then were excitable, but were slower to excite their neighbors (i.e. they went through a "relative refractory period"). Propagation was simulated by having the excitable but not excited neighbors become excited after a specified time delay. This delay was increased during the relative refractory period. The "action potential duration" (or more precisely the refractory periods) could be varied from cell to cell. An "atrium" was created as a flat sheet of cells. "Refractory periods," "conduction velocities," and tissue size were scaled to match the properties found in their prior studies of canine atrial fibrillation [18].

Moe et al. stimulated cells within this model and largely recapitulated their findings from dogs: (i) stimulation at slow rates created organized radial waves of propagation; (ii) stimulation at faster rates could not be conducted 1 : 1 and therefore created wave break. With the full visibility of cell excitation provided by the model, they were also able to see that (i) the area of "turbulence" spread outward from the initiation site and eventually spread to the entire tissue; (ii) self-sustained multiple meandering reentrant waves could be produced; and (iii) the ability to sustain "fibrillation" was related to tissue size, conduction velocity, and refractory period. They even recapitulated the "narrow channel acts like AV node His-Purkinje system" experiments of Garrey. These studies did more than reproduce their canine studies, however. They were additive, in that they demonstrated more definitively that multi-wavelet reentry can drive fibrillation. In the model there could be no ectopic foci (they were not programmed into the "rules") and they had complete knowledge of how activation spread (unlike in the canine heart). They were therefore able to determine that fibrillation was perpetuated by moving reentrant circuits in the absence of any focal driver. Much to their credit, they did not claim that this study proved that multi-wavelet reentry was *the* mechanism of AF, but simply that self-perpetuating, spatially dynamic functional reentry was a viable mechanism of fibrillation.

Numerous human epicardial mapping studies have subsequently been performed on patients with AF. In 1994, Maurits Allessie's group mapped the epicardial right atrium (RA) with 244 electrodes[8] during induced AF in patients undergoing surgery for Wolf Parkinson White (WPW) syndrome. In this study they characterize AF as varying in complexity based upon activation patterns. They suggest that these activation patterns reflect different underlying AF mechanisms: the most organized indicating a single, spatially fixed source with fibrillatory conduction, while the most complex, they postulate, was indicative of multi-wavelet reentry [20].

The following year, Janse mapped "ventricular fibrillation" in a two-dimensional (2D) sheet of epicardial swine ventricular tissue. Three different drivers of fibrillation were observed: (i) multiple wavelet reentry; (ii) two independent wandering reentrant waves; and (iii) a single wandering reentrant wave [21]. Once again, this suggested that identification of changing activation pattern alone is insufficient to determine the arrhythmia's mechanism. The group at UCLA studied ventricular fibrillation (VF) in detail. Mapping of canine ventricles was performed with 509 bipolar electrodes.[9] Meticulous manual (and subsequently automated) activation mapping suggested that fibrillation started as very rapid organized counter-rotating functional circuits (initiated by double extra stimuli). After a brief period, the reentry cores meandered and interacted with each other. The researchers commented: "The VF is maintained and *self-perpetuated* by the continuous regeneration of reentrant wave fronts. The mechanism by which reentry is regenerated is *related to the collision of the wavelets, which result in wave breaks. Tissue mass reduction* by cutting away portions of myocardium results in *decreased* dynamic *complexity and conversion* of VF *to VT* [ventricular tachycardia]" [22] (emphasis added).

Conclusions drawn about the mechanisms that drive fibrillation are

---

[8] 0.3 mm diameter, 2.25 mm interelectrode spacing.

[9] 0.4 mm diameter, 0.5 mm interelectrode spacing.

always subject to the potential error introduced as a result of inadequacies of mapping. This is a subject addressed later in the book, but cannot be ignored in a discussion of postulated mechanisms for fibrillation. One can always wonder whether data points (electrode locations) were too far apart such that the finer details of activation were missed, and inaccurate conclusions were drawn regarding underlying wave direction. Also, unless mapping was performed everywhere at once, one is always left wondering whether something critical was occurring outside of the mapped area. There is, however, evidence unrelated to map accuracy that allows one to deduce that multi-wavelet reentry (in the absence of a focal source) can drive fibrillation. This evidence relates to the **mass hypothesis**.

The mass hypothesis of atrial fibrillation

As already noted, the idea that AF could have a disseminated driver was first postulated *before* any mapping was performed. In Garrey's early studies, it was a fact that fibrillation depended not only upon the area of a piece of tissue, but also upon its width. If fibrillation were driven in these studies by a focal source, then at least *sometimes* the focal source would end up on the smaller piece cut from fibrillating tissue. Size should not matter.[10] It must be conceded here that if a focal source is reentrant, that source would require that the circuit not be interrupted and, as such, cutting a piece of tissue *through the circuit* would terminate the rhythm. However, that would be true *only* at the site that happens to hold the focal driver, not just any site.

James cox: Leveraging the mass hypothesis

The therapeutic implications of the mass hypothesis were appreciated by James Cox. He studied activation during fibrillation in (i) a canine model of atrial fibrillation induced by mitral regurgitation and (ii) in humans who presented for surgical treatment of WPW.[11] In both, he performed epicardial multi-electrode mapping [23]. These maps revealed multiple simultaneous reentrant circuits, particularly in the left atrium. They concluded from their findings that "The presence of macro-reentrant circuits and the absence of either micro-reentrant circuits or evidence of atrial automaticity suggests that

---

[10] A focal source of triggered firing or abnormal automaticity would not have significant tissue size constraints. A focal *reentrant* source (spatially stable rotor or micro-reentry) would require a very small or minimal tissue size.

[11] In whom AF was induced with pacing.

atrial fibrillation should be amenable to surgical ablation."

Having noted that reentrant circuits often remained stationary for periods as short as 200 ms [24], Cox concluded that treatment of fibrillation could not be map guided; rather, he felt that he would need to choose a lesion set that "made it impossible for the atrium to fibrillate at all" [24]. Shortly thereafter, he conceived the creation of a "**maze**" of linear scars that allowed propagation from the sinus node to the AV node (and all atrial myocytes), but were spaced closely enough to "prevent the development of macro-reentrant circuits anywhere in the atria" [24]. In an interesting plot twist, Allessie (ultimately a major figure in the atrial fibrillation story) was visiting Cox's lab during the follow-up clinic visit of the first maze procedure patient, and was the one to "document that the patient was in normal sinus rhythm with no medications" [24].

The maze procedure works. In one large study of the cut-and-sew Cox-maze III,[12] 198 patients (113 paroxysmal and 85 persistent/long-standing persistent) were followed for 5.4 ± 2.9 years. Of the 112 who underwent surgery for AF alone, 96% were in sinus rhythm with or without anti-arrhythmic medication and 80% were in sinus rhythm off anti-arrhythmics [25]. Subsequently, a study of 282 patients undergoing the Cox-maze IV[13] (118 paroxysmal, 28 persistent, and 135 long-standing persistent) found 89% in sinus rhythm with or without anti-arrhythmics and 78% in sinus rhythm off anti-arrhythmics at 12-month follow-up [26]. It is hard to believe that the maze would consistently work with a mechanism other than multi-wavelet reentry. One can imagine that *sometimes* the maze lesion set inadvertently cuts directly through a focal driver site, but surely not in ~80% of cases. You might argue that the maze lesion set quarantines a focal driver site from the remainder of the atria (e.g. by isolating the pulmonary veins). However, that would result in a focal rhythm within the isolated region (albeit no longer driving

---

[12] The initial maze surgeries involved literally slicing transmurally and sewing, to create linear, non-conducting scars. Subsequent procedures have employed radiofrequency (RF) and/or cryo energy to create lesions.

[13] The Cox-maze III consisted of left atria appendectomy, isolation of all four pulmonary veins, connection of the vein line to the mitral annulus and to the appendage line, an intercaval line, a connection of the intercaval line to the tricuspid annulus, and a right atrial appendectomy. The Cox-maze IV replaced much of the cut-and-sew lesions with cryo and RF and eliminated the pulmonary vein to left atrial appendage (LAA) line, eliminated the right atrial appendectomy, and added a line from the superior tricuspid annulus to the right atrial appendage and from the right atrial appendage toward the superior vena cava (SVC), ending approximately 2 cm before the intercaval line.

the atria); this is not what we see. You could argue that the maze is interfering with fibrillatory conduction (not the actual driver of fibrillation), but this would simply convert fibrillation into an organized atrial tachycardia. Perhaps the maze lesion set alters atrial autonomic inputs, resulting in prolongation of wave length, precluding rotors, and/or perhaps eliminating triggered firing? After all, it has been clear for a very long time that parasympathetic tone can decrease wave length and increase the propensity for fibrillation. This has been the impetus for a large body of work attempting to alter atrial autonomic inputs (e.g. ablation of ganglionated plexi) as a stand-alone or adjunctive treatment for fibrillation. However, the mixed results of these attempts (like much in the AF therapy literature) suggest that the mechanism is complex and, very likely, is not the same in all patients. At the very least, there appears to be reason to believe that multi-wavelet reentry *can* cause AF.

What does the physiology of propagation suggest about AF?

Principles of propagation: Implications for fibrillation

It is easier to understand the physiology of AF if we break it into its components. First we'll explore moving functional circuits (multi-wavelet reentry), in the absence of stationary drivers. Next we'll delve into focal drivers (rotors and micro-reentry). Only after we've considered the physiology of each of these separately will we try to put it all together and think through the more complex case in which multiple driver types co-exist and (preview of coming attractions) interact.

Multi-wavelet reentry

In Part I, we discussed what the principles of propagation tell us about functional reentry: that wave break can lead to a curved wave front, source-sink mismatch, and rotation. We also explored the impact that wave length being greater than path length has at the core of a rotor. The wave tip collides with its own tail and propagates along it, causing meander. While there is rotation around the central core (meandering or not), waves propagate outward from the center of rotation (Figure 23). If these "arms" encounter obstacles to conduction (e.g. areas of heterogeneous refractoriness), there can be wave break and possibly new rotor formation. It is easy to see how functional circuits moving across tissue that has intrinsic heterogeneity (of action potential duration, conduction velocity, and tissue architecture) will create further heterogeneity (via dyssyn-

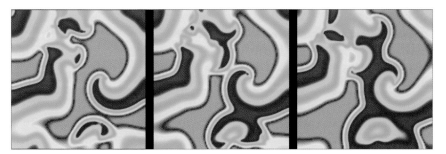

Figure 23 **Multiwavelet reentry**. What begins as an organized rotor degenerates into multi-wavelet reentry when the spiral arms of the rotor encounter refractory tissue and break. New rotors are formed, which in turn develop wave breaks. Here we see the evolution of multiple rotors (three snapshots separated by 100 ms each) with collision and wave breaks in several locations. *Source*: Reproduced with permission from Visible Electrophysiology LLC.

chrony). Circuits with a propensity to meander (WL > PL) meander more still when interacting with other waves [10]. Soon there is dynamic, shifting, self-perpetuating functional reentry: multi-wavelet reentry. This process will be perpetuated unless all the reentrant circuits are interrupted.

Once initiated, how does multi-wavelet reentry ever stop? Reentry termination requires circuit transection. Transection must be complete (from the core to an outer boundary). This is as true for a functional circuit as it is for a structural circuit. But how do the moving circuits of multi-wavelet reentry get transected? The very fact that circuits move provides the answer: *moving circuits collide with boundaries and transect themselves* [3, 10, 27–31]. As it turns out, this relatively simplistic

notion has wide-ranging implications that help to explain the mass hypothesis, anti-arrhythmic drug action, and electrical remodeling, and that point the way toward the development of effective ablation strategies.

Movement of circuits (more specifically circuit cores) is largely random, and hence *where* they will be is a probabilistic phenomenon. Probability plays a critical role in many areas of science, but is not something that we spend much time thinking about in electrophysiology, so it can take some getting used to before you have an intuitive feel for its implications in the treatment of AF.

If the core of a circuit is stationary, the probability of meandering into a boundary is… zero. Thus the probabilistic formulation doesn't apply to all mechanisms of fibrillation:[14] it applies only when meandering functional circuits participate in driving AF (multi-wavelet reentry). Not surprisingly, treatment depends upon mechanism. Let's begin by discussing the treatment of moving circuits.

Multi-wavelet reentry: the probabilistic formulation

Moving circuits transect themselves. To understand this, think about it from a physical perspective. A reentrant wave propagates continuously, because it continuously encounters excitable cells. This is why circuit transection is the treatment for reentry: when the wave front encounters no excitable cells, propagation ceases. To apply this to moving circuits, we simply consider what happens when a moving circuit collides with a tissue boundary. The boundary (e.g. a valve ring) is where one runs out of excitable cells. So, what part of the circuit must run into the boundary in order to transect the circuit? The core. Picture what happens when the core comes close to, but doesn't quite reach, the boundary (Figure 24). A path remains for propagation around the core (i.e.

there is still a circuit).[15] If the core itself reaches the boundary, every cell in the wave front collides with the boundary.

Collision probability

If termination is caused by core versus boundary collisions, what does that imply for the relative capacity of a particular heart to maintain multi-wavelet reentry? In the simplest formulation, we can consider the answer to this question in a scenario where a core *moves randomly*.[16] The probability of a core hitting a boundary relates to the ratio of the number of places it could meander to without hitting a boundary relative to the number of boundary locations. Thus, collision probability is related to atrial shape: shape determines the ratio of places a randomly moving core could go *without* hitting a boundary versus the number where it *would* hit a boundary. The surface area is a quantification of "the number of places without a boundary," and the perimeter is the number of places that are on a boundary.

---

[14] Actually, as I will discuss later, because of the chaotic nature of fibrillatory conduction, even focal drivers of AF are subject to probability. But details of probability's role differ between multi-wavelet reentry and focal drivers.

[15] A core that doesn't reach the boundary is analogous to an incomplete (non-transecting) ablation line.

[16] Equally likely to move in any direction at any moment.

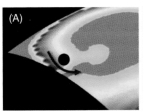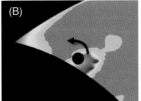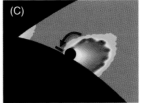

Figure 24 **Core misses boundary**. (A) When a meandering core comes near to, but does not touch, a boundary, a path remains for propagation between the core and the boundary (arrow). (B) Reentry continues around the core. (C) When the core hits the boundary, there are no excitable cells and wave annihilation will occur. *Source*: Reproduced with permission from Visible Electrophysiology LLC.

With this as our model, it is clear that a circle, for example, would support fibrillation better than a star. In the circle, the ratio of surface area (places that are *not* on a boundary) to boundary length is high, whereas in the star the ratio is much lower: most of the places to which a core could meander in a star-shaped tissue would result in a boundary collision and annihilation.

Episode duration and collision probability

There is an inverse relationship between the probability of boundary collision and the average duration of an episode of AF: if collision probability is high, on average, episodes will be short. But atrial tissue can simultaneously support more than one circuit. In the presence of multiple circuits, fibrillation will not terminate until *all* circuits are annihilated. If only one or a few circuits are annihilated, the wave fronts emanating from the remaining circuits can break and form new circuits. Mathematically, the probability of *all* rotors colliding with boundaries equals the probability of *each* rotor colliding, *raised to the power* of the number of rotors. This means that having multiple rotors very markedly decreases the probability of spontaneous AF termination, and hence is associated with a longer average episode duration. Wave length determines the number of rotors that can fit on the tissue at one time, and hence has a large impact on the capacity of the atrium to support fibrillation (Figure 25) [32, 33].

Quantifying the propensity to perpetuate multi-wavelet reentry

We've now reduced the question of how long an episode of multi-wavelet reentry will last (on average) to the less complex question: What determines

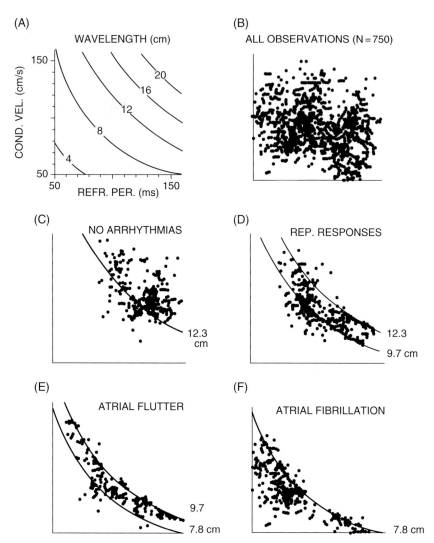

Figure 25 Wave length and inducible rhythms. (A) Wave length (lines) is revealed by plotting refractory period (x-axis) against conduction velocity (y-axis). Paced beats were delivered during various combinations of refractory period and conduction velocity (B). When type of rhythm induced is potted on the wave length plot (C–F), it becomes clear that wave length influences the rhythms the tissue is able to support. No arrhythmia (C), non-sustained reentry (D), atrial flutter (E), and atrial fibrillation (F). *Source*: Reproduced with permission from [33].

the probability of spontaneous termination of multi-wavelet reentry? Since this probability is based upon the various parameters that influence collision, we have a means to quantify the capacity of a chamber to support multi-wavelet reentry. The probability of a *single circuit colliding* with a boundary is *related to the area to boundary length ratio*, and the *number of circuits* is *inversely related* to the tissue *wave length*.

In our lab, we performed a series of computational studies to investigate how well the probabilistic formulation could predict the behavior of multi-wavelet reentry. Based upon the principles just discussed, we formulated a metric for the capacity to support fibrillation, which we call the fibrillogenicity index (Fb):[17]

$$Fb = A/(BL * APD * CV)$$

where Fb = fibrillogenicity index, A = area, BL = boundary length, APD = action potential duration, and CV = conduction velocity. To test our hypothesis, we created a large number of tissues, varying each of the parameters that contribute to fibrillogenicity (area, boundary length, action potential duration, and conduction velocity).[18] We used flat, 2D sheets of cells, but we could have used tissues with thickness and tissues with more complex shapes (e.g. atrial anatomy). By choosing a relatively simplistic model, we were able to generate and test a very large range of tissue parameters and could more easily vary a single parameter at a time. Having created these tissues, we induced multi-wavelet reentry (via burst pacing) and measured episode duration as a function of the components of the fibrillogenicity index.

Figure 26 shows the average half-life of multi-wavelet reentry episodes [34]. The first plot (Figure 26A) demonstrates that episode duration increases as the area to boundary length ratio increases. The second plot (Figure 26B) shows a decrease of episode duration with increasing APD (and, hence, increased wave length). The third plot (Figure 26C) is where things get interesting. You can see that as intercellular resistance increases (decreasing conduction velocity and therefore decreasing

---

[17] In 1964, Moe did his study of AF in a computer model. He discussed the potential for using a "fibrillation number" to characterize the probability of "turbulent" propagation. His number was LT/K, where L is a length that characterizes the "model" (the tissue), T is conduction time (inverse of conduction velocity), and K is a "materials" constant [19].

[18] In our model, conduction velocity isn't a parameter, it is an emergent result of the action potential upstroke velocity and intercellular resistance (among other things). In this study we varied intercellular resistance to alter conduction velocity.

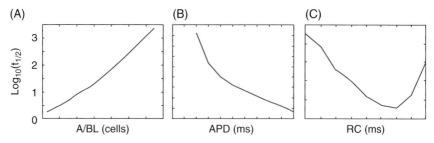

Figure 26 Multi-wavelet reentry as a function of fibrillogenicity indices. (A) Duration increases with area/boundary length ratio (A/BL). (B) Duration decreases as action potential duration (APD) increases. (C) Duration first decreases and then increases as resistance is increased (RC – resistance and capacitance). Log scale: i.e. 1 = 10, 2 = 100, and 3 = 1000 seconds. *Source*: Modified with permission from [34].

wave length), there is initially a decrease in episode duration, but as you increase resistance further, episode duration begins to *increase*![19] The first plot, second plot, and beginning of the third plot are all consistent with the predictions of the probabilistic formulation. The far-right portion of the third plot is not consistent. We dug deeper.

We examined the activation patterns during the rhythms we had induced over the entire range of tissue properties. We found that propagation behavior changes as tissue properties change. This is not surprising: What else would propagation behavior depend upon? The rhythms generated could be broken into three categories: almost entirely moving circuits, a mixture of moving and stationary circuits, and mostly stationary circuits. If we look at all episodes of fibrillation together (regardless of circuit movement) and try to correlate episode duration with the fibrillogenicity index, the correlation is poor – $r^2 = 0.42$ (Figure 27A). But when we separate episodes by type of fibrillation, we see that the poor correlation is due to the presence of spatially stable rotors. This makes sense; after all, the probability of a stationary rotor meandering into a boundary is zero. The correlation between episode duration and fibrillogenicity index is very good once we consider only moving circuits – $r^2 = 0.82$ (Figure 27B) [34]. The fibrillogenicity index captures the parameters that determine the probability of spontaneous termination of moving circuits sufficiently well to allow prediction of

---

[19] Excitable gap was increased such that the number of waves on the tissue decreased, reducing episode duration.

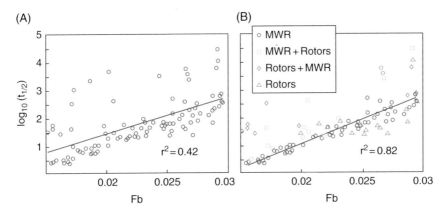

Figure 27 Duration of fibrillation vs. fibrillogenicity (Fb) index. (A) Circles indicate the Fb index and duration of all episodes. (B) When episodes are divided by type of fibrillation, correlation is much improved ($r^2 = 0.82$). MWR, multi-wavelet reentry. *Source*: Modified with permission from [34].

episode duration. AF does not always comprise moving circuits and therefore the fibrillogenicity index is not sufficient to characterize all fibrillation; more on this later.

The probabilistic formulation fits with some of the things we know about AF. Early in the course of fibrillation, episodes are relatively short lived, terminating spontaneously. Episode durations vary from episode to episode based upon the whims of probabilistic phenomena. But AF tends to get worse over time (less likely to spontaneously terminate and therefore longer average episode durations). There is an expression, "atrial fibrillation begets atrial fibrillation," which refers to the negative feedback loop in which

AF itself causes electrophysiological changes in the atria that promote fibrillation. These changes, termed remodeling, tend to alter the probability of core versus boundary collisions. Area to boundary length ratio increases; atrial dilation causes a greater increase of surface area than of boundary length. Simultaneously, wave length is decreased, because changes in the expression of ion channels decrease refractory period and conduction velocity. Interstitial fibrosis compounds the decrease in conduction velocity. The combined impact of increased area to boundary length ratio and decreased wave length is a decreased probability of core versus boundary collisions (i.e. spontaneous termination probability

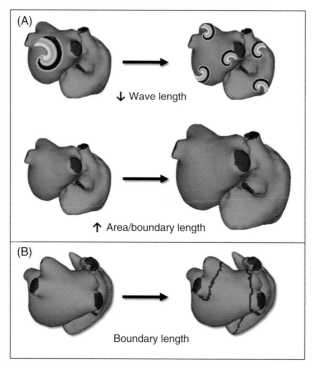

Figure 28 Fibrillogenicity index, remodeling, and ablation. (A) (top) As atrial fibrillation (AF) progresses, wave length decreases (due to decreased action potential duration and slowed conduction velocity). As a result, a greater number of circuits can fit on the atria, reducing the probability of all circuits being annihilated. (bottom) Atria dilate as AF progresses, increasing area more than boundary length. Once again, the result is reduced probability of *each* circuit colliding with a boundary and being annihilated. (B) The area/boundary length ratio can be decreased by *adding* boundaries via linear ablation, thereby increasing the probability of core vs. boundary collision and AF termination. *Source*: Reproduced with permission from Visible Electrophysiology LLC.

diminishes and episode duration increases) (Figure 28A).[20]

---

[20] There's more to it than simply increasing the area to boundary length ratio and decreasing wave length. As we will discuss soon, remodeling can promote rotor stability, which obviously decreases the probability of meandering into a boundary.

The probabilistic formulation also jibes with the way in which atrial fibrillation responds to anti-arrhythmic medications. Compare the following: when we give adenosine during orthodromic reciprocating tachycardia, AV nodal conduction blocks, and tachycardia *immediately* terminates.[21] In contrast, when we give anti-arrhythmics to an AF patient, fibrillation does not terminate immediately. We have simply increased the probability of spontaneous termination: it takes a variable amount of time before atrial fibrillation actually terminates (if at all). The same is true for the impact of ablation on AF: the goal is to increase the probability of spontaneous termination (Figure 28B). Acute termination is much less meaningful than the impact of ablation on the *capacity to support fibrillation*. Ideally, ablation makes the probability of spontaneous termination so high that episodes effectively cannot persist beyond a matter of seconds.

This all makes plenty of sense for moving circuits. But there is an obvious question that remains thus far unanswered: How does atrial fibrillation, if driven by *stationary* circuits, ever spontaneously terminate? Once again, the physiology of propagation/ reentry tells us: the circuit(s) that drive fibrillation must be interrupted. Thus the question becomes: How are *stationary* circuits spontaneously transected?

There are several means by which stationary circuits can spontaneously terminate. To begin with, the *fact* of

spontaneous termination should not be surprising: all sorts of spatially stable reentrant rhythms spontaneously terminate (e.g. orthodromic reciprocating tachycardia, atrial flutter). Termination can be achieved with (i) an appropriately timed premature beat; (ii) an increase in wave length (greater than path length); (iii) sufficiently decreased excitability in a region of slow conduction (causing failure to excite/block); or (iv) lift-off and meandering of the circuit into a boundary (which causes transection) [35].

Because stationary drivers can be terminated by an appropriately timed external wave, it is not surprising that the chaotic and randomly timed waves of fibrillatory conduction can cause termination. Due to the random nature of fibrillatory conduction, termination of stationary drivers is a probabilistic phenomenon as well.

Predicting the impact of ablation

We've discussed the physiology of propagation and how various parameters relate to the likelihood of spontaneous multi-wavelet reentry termination. Can we now use this understanding to *prospectively* determine how a particular ablation lesion distribution will alter the likelihood of spontaneous termination (i.e. to predict the efficacy of an ablation lesion set)?

---

[21] The probability of termination is either 0 (AV node conducts) or 1 (AV node blocks).

Fibrillogenicity index and predicting ablation impact

The power of the fibrillogenicity index lies in its ability to (i) quantify the capacity of a tissue to sustain multi-wavelet reentry and (ii) calculate the impact of an intervention that alters area/boundary length ratio or wave length. The fibrillogenicity index is not exact. It does not account for all of the parameters that influence multi-wavelet reentry duration, and hence two tissues with different capacities to support multi-wavelet reentry could have the same fibrillogenicity index.[22] It is, however, an excellent example of "pretty good" being far better than nothing at all. Figure 29 demonstrates this value. In a series of tissues with different fibrillogenicity indices (and as you can see, corresponding average episode durations), one can choose an arbitrary desired value for average duration and then add linear ablation to alter the A/BL ratio until the fibrillogenicity index falls below that threshold. When we ran simulations of these tissues, the average episode duration remained on the curve produced by the fibrillogenicity index [36]. A similar calculation could be performed for alterations of wave length (e.g. due to anti-arrhythmic medications).

What the fibrillogenicity index doesn't account for: There are many factors that are not taken into account in the fibrillogenicity index. It ignores the role of tissue architecture, tissue thickness (and endocardial/epicardial dissociation), and heterogeneity, and, perhaps most significantly, it does not apply in the setting where all circuits are stationary.[23] This does not mean that it has no value, but in order to make use of a tool (even an analytic one), you must understand what it is good for and what it isn't.

Assuming for a moment that the fibrillogenicity index can tell you *how much* ablation is required, does it matter where the ablation lesion(s) are delivered? How about whether the ablation is delivered as one long line or two shorter lines? Should the line be straight or shaped like a fork or an antenna? How do we decide?

To address this question, let's consider *how* ablation lesions diminish the capacity of the tissue to support multi-wavelet reentry. Given that ablation lesions exert their anti-fibrillatory effect via increasing the probability of core versus boundary collisions, one

---

[22] Its accuracy is also mitigated by the extent to which focal drivers contribute to maintenance of fibrillation.

[23] For a discussion of optimizing ablation lesion distribution in the setting of stationary drivers or mixed stationary and dynamic drivers, see Section 2.3.6.1.2.

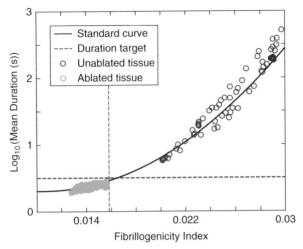

Figure 29 Prospectively predicting ablation impact. Duration of multi-wavelet reentry is plotted against the fibrillogenicity index (Fb) for a range of tissue parameters (circles: red unablated, green ablated tissues). The points fall along the theoretical line (blue) relating Fb to duration. The total length of ablation was calculated to bring Fb below an arbitrary threshold (black dashed line) in hopes of reducing duration below the duration threshold (red dashed line). Following ablation (green circles), duration plotted vs. Fb index accurately predicted post-ablation duration. *Source*: Modified with permission from [34].

can conclude that the effectiveness of any given distribution of ablation lesions corresponds to the extent to which the probability of such collisions has been increased.

We performed a series of modeling experiments in which we quantified how often waves passed over each location of a tissue during multi-wavelet reentry. We tested how *ablation lesion distribution* affected this wave distribution.

Figure 30 represents three rectangular sheets of cells, each with ablation lesions distributed differently. The colors represent the number of times any wave front propagated over each cell/location per second. Red sites contained a wave front 20 times in a second, while blue had only 10 waves. What's interesting is how the presence of an ablation line influences the number of waves that propagate in the lesion's vicinity. First, note that fewer waves are seen in the corners of the tissue. Why do you think this is? You can also see that there are fewer waves adjacent to the ablation lines. This is because waves in these locations are more likely to be annihilated. There is yet one more thing that stands out in the wave map. There are

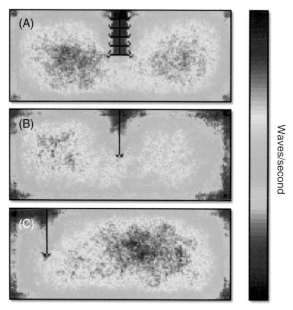

Figure 30 Wave–boundary interactions. Color-coded plot of the number of times a wave passed over each cell in the tissue during multi-wavelet reentry. Black lines are ablation lines. (A) With an "antennae"-shaped ablation, very few waves reach the inner portions of the ablation. (B) With an ablation line in the middle of the tissue, there is fairly uniform wave distribution. (C) When the ablation line is moved toward the left side of the tissue, fewer waves access the side of the ablation facing the tissue edge. Note that wave number is reduced along the tissue edges, particularly in the corners. *Source*: Reproduced with permission from Visible Electrophysiology LLC.

consistently fewer waves in the region between closely spaced ablation lines (Figure 30). Picture what a wave in these regions looks like. It is likely that any wave that enters the space between the ablation lines will have both of its wave ends anchored to the ablation lines (Figure 31). When this occurs, there is no access of the wave front to cells that recover from refractoriness (behind the wave tail), so the wave will inevitably be extinguished. At first glance, this seems like the perfect ablation lesion set design: effectively a "trap" where waves can get in, but they can't get out. This is absolutely true; however, we are not simply seeking ablation lines that will result in circuit annihilation when a wave front comes into contact with it – we are looking for an ablation lesion set that has maximum *efficiency* (i.e. the largest anti-fibrillatory impact *per individual ablation point*). The "wave trap" configuration is effective, but not efficient. The arms of the wave

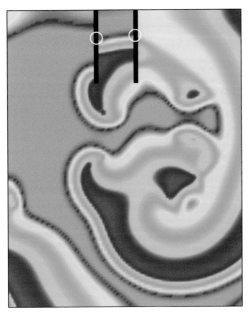

Figure 31 Wave interactions with closely spaced ablation lines. During multi-wavelet reentry, circuit cores rarely enter the space between closely spaced ablation lines. Instead, spiral arms enter this space. Both wave ends (white circles) are on the same boundary and therefore reentry is not possible; annihilation of entering waves results. *Source*: Reproduced with permission from Visible Electrophysiology LLC.

trap make it less likely that a core will reach the innermost portion of the ablation line.[24] The arms effectively

shield some of the ablation lesion, rendering them *less* likely to collide with a core.[25]

Similarly, look at the number of waves that interact with the sides of the straight ablation lines (Figure 30). When the line is in the center of the tissue, there is the same number of wave interactions on both of its sides. Compare this with the ablation line that is near the edge of the tissue. Here, there are more wave–line interactions

---

[24] If you think about it, this is why fibrillation cannot be directly transmitted through a narrow gap (Garrey experiment). Cores can't get through, so the far side is focally activated like during pre-excitation. I say fibrillation cannot be *directly* transmitted, but if the waves emerge faster than the longest refractory period on the far side, they can *induce* fibrillation. This is why accessory pathways with a short refractory period increase the risk of sudden death. AF isn't directly transmitted to the ventricle; rapid excitation at the ventricular insertion site of the pathway acts like burst pacing to induce fibrillation.

[25] Less likely than the most exposed portions of the ablation line.

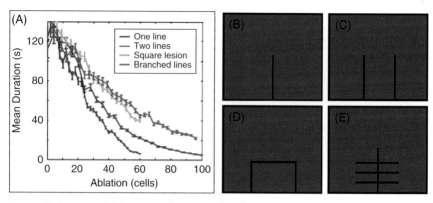

Figure 32 Impact of ablation on duration of multi-wavelet reentry. (A) Mean duration of multi-wavelet reentry plotted against number of ablated cells for different lesion distributions. Impact per ablated cell for one line (blue), two lines (red), square (green), and antennae-shaped (pink) lesions. (B) Single line, (C) two lines, (D) square lesion, and (E) "antennae"-shaped lesions. Note: The square lesion "quarantines" the tissue within the ablation from the remainder of the tissue. This reduces the boundary length compared with ablation lines that have both sides exposed to the tissue. It also reduces the area of the tissue, hence it changes the area to boundary length ratio via both area and boundary length. *Source*: Modified with permission from [36].

on the side of the line away from the tissue edge. This is because the line itself (along with the tissue edge) blocks some of the waves from reaching the far side of the line. Quantifying *wave* versus boundary interactions is not a direct measure of the ability to terminate moving circuits (for this we would need to examine circuit *core* versus boundary interactions).

In order to directly test the relative impact of ablation with different shapes, we measured average duration. Figure 32 directly demonstrates the efficiency of ablation (change in multi-wavelet reentry duration *per ablated cell*). A single line is more efficient than two lines and branched lines are least

efficient. Why do you suppose the square lesion is inefficient?[26]

We also assessed the impact of line *position* on average episode duration (Figure 33A) [36]. When the ablation line is in the center of the tissue, the episode duration is shortest. As you move the line toward either of the edges, episode duration increases. As the line

---

[26] Answer: Because only one side is exposed to circuits. Therefore, each lesion point is at most half as effective as a lesion which does not "quarantine" any tissue. Its overall impact on multi-wavelet reentry is complex, because quarantine reduces area, which also alters the area to boundary length ratio. In a clinical setting, posterior wall isolation reduces area *and*, in some cases, eliminates drivers.

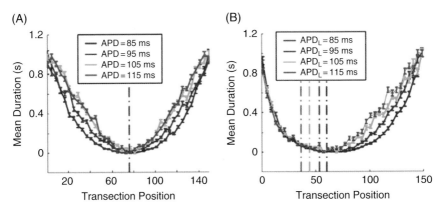

Figure 33 **Effect of ablation location on multi-wavelet reentry duration**. Duration of multi-wavelet reentry plotted against location of a vertical ablation line on a rectangular sheet of tissue (e.g. see Figure 34B). (A) In homogeneous tissue, ablation in the center of the tissue (red dashed line) has the greatest impact on episode duration. As the line moves toward either side of the tissue, episode duration increases (i.e. ablation is less effective). Y-axis duration, x-axis ablation position measured in mm from the left edge of the tissue (tissue width 150 mm). Line color corresponds to tissues with different average action potential durations (APDs) indicated. (B) The same plot but on heterogeneous tissue, where the left half of the tissue has a shorter APD (85 ms) vs. the longer right side (APDs indicated). As the gradient in APD increases, the most effective ablation location shifts further into the short wave length region. *Source*: Reproduced with permission from [36].

moves closer to one of the tissue's edges, the total number of wave lesion interactions decreases. In the very center of the tissue, both sides of the line have maximum wave exposure [36].

Predicting the impact of ablation in heterogeneous tissue

The modeling studies described earlier were performed in homogeneous tissues (there was no regional variation of APD or intercellular resistance).[27] How

does the analysis change if the waves/cores are not uniformly distributed on the tissue? In a simple set of computational experiments, we created rectangular tissues in which one half of the tissue had a shorter wave length than the other half. What effect do you suppose this had on the location at which an ablation line was most efficient? Figure 33B shows the efficiency curves for ablation in these tissues. When there were more waves on the left side of the tissue, an ablation line closer to that side was more efficient than one at the tissue's center [36]. The same was

---

[27] And therefore there was a homogeneous distribution of circuit cores.

(A)

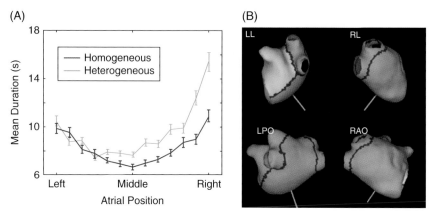

(B)

Figure 34 Impact of ablation position in left atrial geometry. A standard left atrial maze lesion set (pulmonary vein isolation, roof, and left mitral isthmus lines) was performed. We then assessed the impact of a transecting ablation (using a *septal* mitral line) that either divided the tissue area in half or was closer to one side or the other. (A) Plot indicates episode duration as a function of line position. When the tissue had homogeneous action potential duration, the optimal ablation position was in the middle of the tissue area (blue line). When the tissue had a short wave length patch on the left side (yellow patch), the optimal ablation location was closer to the left side of the tissue (green line). (B) Views: left lateral (LL), right lateral (RL), left posterior oblique (LPO), right anterior oblique (RAO). *Source*: Modified with permission from [36].

true when the analogous experiment was done on the more complex simulated landscape of atrial-shaped tissue (Figure 34) [36].

Geometric optimization
We've established that the impact of ablation on multi-wavelet reentry varies with ablation location. We've also seen that location matters *because* of its impact on the probability of wave versus boundary interactions.[28] The question remains: How

do we predict precisely *where* ablation will maximize these collisions? In the earlier examples, the efficacy of ablation shifted toward the side of the tissue where circuit density was higher. But, how do we know *how much* to shift our line toward the higher circuit density region? If we go too far, we increase the probability of collision with cores on the left, but we decrease the probability of colliding with cores on the right. Where is the "sweet spot"?

It is also far simpler to calculate collision probability in a rectangle, with a geometrically simplistic circuit

---

[28] And presumably on core versus boundary, although we did not directly demonstrate this.

core distribution (i.e. half the tissue). Determining the same thing in complex atrial architecture and with a complex circuit core distribution is far more challenging.

Modeling core versus boundary collision as a random walk

In order to approach the "sweet spot" question, we can strip away all the details of multi-wavelet reentry and wave dynamics. We simply model random movement in the abstract to investigate the most *efficient* distribution of ablation lesions.[29] A "random walk" refers to a system that *behaves like* "a drunk person walking" – at any moment they could take a step in any direction, regardless of the direction of their prior step. This is far from a precise description of the movement of circuit cores in multi-wavelet reentry. But it does capture some of the macroscopic features of multi-wavelet reentry: *overall* cores move in largely unpredictable and chaotic directions.

When such a core is likely to hit a boundary is a probabilistic question. By this I mean that because the core could move in any direction at any time, we can't know exactly what it will do at a particular time, and therefore we certainly can't know exactly when it will "happen to" collide with a boundary.

As we will see, using the mathematical properties of a random walk allows us to make predictions about the median duration of an episode of multi-wavelet reentry for a given tissue.

Let's consider the simplest version of a random walk to get a feel for how this is relevant to AF. Imagine that the "walk" occurs on a one dimensional number line: we start at 0 and with each step have a 50/50 chance of going in the forward (positive) or backward (negative) direction (Figure 35). We will ultimately extrapolate this to a meandering core starting somewhere in the atrium, and derive the probability of its hitting a boundary within a certain time frame. This has the advantage of reducing our *physiological* question (movement of functional reentrant circuits) into a *geometric* question (a "walk" over a 2D surface) in which we need only consider the size and shape of the atrium,[30] the distribution of moving cores, and the regional rates of core movement.

---

[29] Note: The study presented here has not yet been submitted for publication and therefore has not undergone peer review.

[30] In order to do this, we need to "discretize" the atria (break the surface and boundaries into a finite number of specific locations). This is not actually so unrealistic, in that cores can only be found at the junctions between cells (a discrete/finite quantity).

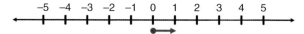

Figure 35 One-dimensional random walk. The number line represents the "tissue." The walker (red point) starts in the center (0) and with each step moves either right (arrow) or left based upon a fair coin flip. The edges of the "tissue" are at ± 5.

Let's return to the number-line walker. Knowing the "rules of the game" (one step at a time, 50/50 chance of going in either direction), we can calculate the probability of traveling any distance in any amount of time (number of steps). Specifically, we could ask: What is the number of steps in which there is a 50% probability of reaching the "edge of the tissue"?[31] This tells us how long it will take for half of the "episodes of multi-wavelet reentry" to terminate... *if the core always starts in the middle of the tissue* (0 on the number line). What if the core is only *sometimes* found in the middle, or if the core is more likely to be found in the region between −5 and −1 on the number line? Here's how we could account for those scenarios. We separately calculate the probability of hitting either boundary, starting from *each point* and then, to calculate the overall

probability of termination (accounting for a core that could start at any location), we "weigh" each of these probabilities based upon the likelihood of finding a core at each location. When we do this, we see that the number of steps and the amount of time correlate directly with the distance between the starting point and the boundaries. To find out how we actually calculate these probabilities, see Appendix A.

So, how can we extrapolate this simple 1D formulation to the more complex 3D topology of the atria? If we discretize the atria (Figure 36A), we can calculate the distance from each cell within the atria to each cell on the boundaries of the atria. If we calculate the average of all of these distances,[32] we should have a metric that correlates with the median duration of multi-wavelet reentry *in the setting of uniform core distribution*. If we combine this information with a circuit core density map (which quantifies the relative probability of finding a core at

---

[31] If we know the distance from the middle of a one-dimensional (1D) atrium to the boundary (the same distance in either direction, since we are starting in the middle), this tells us how long it will take until half the episodes of multi-wavelet reentry on this tissue will terminate (core collides with boundary).

[32] I.e. the shortest distance from each location on the tissue to each location on the boundaries.

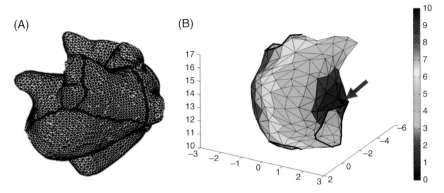

Figure 36 **Initial steps of geometric optimization**. (A) Discretized left atrium (B) color coded by shortest distances from a boundary point (arrow) to each cell. This is repeated for every boundary cell. Discretization can be performed at multiple levels of resolution: (A) is ~5000 cells, (B) is ~350 cells.

each location in the atria), we can weigh the distances associated with each site by the likelihood of finding a core at that location. This should correlate with the median duration of multi-wavelet reentry *in the setting of heterogeneous core distribution.*

It is not particularly useful simply to determine the median duration of multi-wavelet reentry in a particular heart. But it would be very useful if we could use this method to *predict* the median duration of multi-wavelet reentry *if we created a certain ablation lesion distribution.* This would provide a method for predicting the impact of ablation *before* creating lesions. We could test a series of potential lesion sets and determine which would result in the lowest weighted average distance, and hence the shortest median duration of

multi-wavelet reentry. We could then search for the most *efficient* ablation lesion set: the smallest weighted average distance *per ablation* point (i.e. weighted average distance divided by the number of cells ablated – Figure 36B).

We can modify the weighting of average distances formulation to include other factors that will influence collision probability. We could weight paths differently, based upon their direction, if cores are more likely to move in one direction or another. We could also use weighting to account for regional variation in the extent of movement (i.e. variable "step size").[33]

You've likely noticed that I've been talking about ablation of multi-wavelet

---

[33] As we will see later, meander distance can vary regionally.

reentry, not AF (regardless of mechanism). Thus the preceding discussion applies to AF driven by *moving circuits*; what about stationary circuits? Any useful real-world treatment for AF must take into consideration all the *possible* mechanisms for AF. In order to get there, we must first discuss focal drivers of AF.

Focal rotors

Among the postulated mechanisms of fibrillation is that a single, spatially stable, focal source could drive fibrillation: by generating waves at a rate faster than can be conducted 1 : 1 through the chamber, fibrillatory conduction results. A focal driver (regardless of its type) whose cycle length is longer than the longest refractory period in the surrounding tissue will conduct 1 : 1. This would be atrial *tachycardia*, not fibrillation. If, on the other hand, a driver's cycle length is shorter than the refractory period of *some* but not all cells, waves will break at the refractory sites, initiating chaotic, shifting conduction. The intrinsic heterogeneity of varied APDs is exacerbated as cells are excited out of phase with one another, such that irregular conduction, once initiated, will tend to be perpetuated, even if conduction is entirely secondary to the driver.

In 1948, Scherf produced AF in a canine model by applying aconitine to the right atrium [37]. Aconitine injection caused rapid focal firing at the site of injection. When this firing was slow, it was conducted in a 1 : 1 fashion through the atria. When firing was sufficiently rapid, propagation was irregular, causing fibrillation. Scherf noted that when firing was stopped (by cooling the site of injection), fibrillation immediately ceased. When firing resumed (upon relief from cooling), fibrillation resumed as well. This demonstrated that fibrillation *can* be driven from a focal source and that the fibrillatory conduction so produced does not possess the capacity to sustain itself (i.e. in the absence of the driver, fibrillatory conduction ceased).

One of the advantages of this study design is that it allows one to deduce that fibrillation is focally driven *without requiring high-density mapping*. One simply needs to be able to see that activation is irregular (an EKG will suffice) and fulfill Koch's postulates with focal firing.[34]

In 1992, Schuessler's group set out to test the "multiple wavelet hypothesis." They used a perfused and superfused

---

[34] Start rapid firing, start fibrillation. Remove rapid firing, stop fibrillation. Reintroduce rapid firing, reinitiate fibrillation.

portion of the right atrium excised from normal canine hearts [37]. Tissues were approximately 38 cm². They performed high-density bipolar electrogram mapping.[35] Single extra stimuli were delivered in the baseline state and with progressively higher concentrations of acetylcholine in the perfusate.

They mapped propagation during the initial stimulus drive train and with premature stimuli. At baseline, the premature beat conducted more slowly than beats during the slower drive train, there were often areas with functional conduction block during premature stimuli, but there were no instances of reentry. With the addition of low-concentration acetylcholine, premature stimuli produced one or more beats of reentry. These rotated around shifting areas of functional block (i.e. the location of reentry varied from beat to beat). At lower concentrations of acetylcholine, "fibrillation" was never sustained. As acetylcholine concentration increased, they were able to induce sustained fibrillation with single extra stimuli. What's interesting is that when fibrillation was sustained, it was not multi-wavelet reentry. Fibrillation was only sustained when there was a stationary repetitive functional reentrant circuit. These studies clearly demonstrate that fibrillation can be driven by a focal driver and that the driver can be a functional reentrant circuit. The authors noted that their methods favored the initiation of stable rotors: "Any non-reentrant mechanism, such as automaticity or triggered automaticity, would be suppressed by Ach."[36] Moreover, in Moe's demonstration of multi-wavelet reentry "tissue was approximately 158-cm² compared with the 38-cm² piece of atrium used in the present study." The point is that based upon the mass hypothesis, use of a smaller piece of tissue reduced the capacity to support multi-wavelet reentry and therefore, via selection bias, increased the likelihood of observing focal drivers.

In 1990, Jalife's group employed optical mapping[37] of thin slices of sheep ventricular myocardium. They were able to induce sustained rotors and demonstrate that these could be terminated by an appropriately timed premature beat (if it had access to the

---

[35] 250 bipolar pairs, 76 µm diameter silver wire, intrabipolar distance of 200 µm, and interbipolar distance of 5 mm.

[36] Acetylcholine.

[37] In optical mapping, voltage-sensitive dyes perfuse the heart. Waves of excitation are thus *visible* as varying colors traversing the heart in waves.

excitable gap[38]) [38]. In a follow-up study of sheep and canine epicardial ventricular slices, they found that rotors could anchor to small arteries or bands of connective tissue, or could drift and extinguish themselves at the border of the tissue [30]. In these tissues they had created focal rotors with 1 : 1 conduction to the remainder of the tissue (i.e. tachycardia, not fibrillation). Later, in a study which combined computational modeling with optical mapping of ventricular sheets, they showed that, in homogeneous tissue, rotors were stationary and could persist indefinitely [39]. Whereas, in heterogeneous tissue, rotors would drift and terminate against a tissue border. A "pseudo-electrocardiogram"[39] recorded during rotor drift manifested an irregular "QRS," mimicking torsade de pointe. This indicates the possibility of irregular activation (fibrillation) due to meander alone.

The group next demonstrated that in rabbit and sheep ventricles, a rotor whose cycle length is shorter than the longest ventricular refractory period will propagate with fibrillatory conduction. They characterized the behavior of this fibrillatory conduction by identifying and examining phase singularities.[40] The majority of these were short-lived, ~80% lasting less than one rotation (<100 ms) [40]. They terminated when two rotors of opposite chirality merged or when a single rotor meandered into a boundary.

Jalife's group also studied AF in Langendorff-perfused sheep hearts. In this study they established the relationship between the rate of rotors and the *dominant frequency*[41] of pseudo-EKGs (generated from optical data) [41].

Optical mapping provides direct visualization of propagation. An optical map offers a level of data unavailable to clinicians (the voltage-sensitive dyes are toxic, so cannot be used in humans). The investigators therefore examined pseudo-EKGs (because EKGs can easily be obtained clinically). EKGs and electrograms

---

[38] The excitable gap is the space (or time) between the end of refractoriness and before the next excitation. At a specific location the excitable gap refers to a time interval; within a circuit the excitable gap refers to a physical distance (the distance between path length and wave length).

[39] A pseudo-EKG calculates the electrical activity from the entire sheet of tissue.

[40] A phase map plots the distribution of various phases of excitation (i.e. upstroke, plateau, repolarization, and baseline). A phase singularity is a point on this map where all phases meet, in sequence, in one location. A phase singularity therefore represents a discrete rotor core at a particular moment.

[41] Dominant frequency is a measure of the frequency components of a signal; see next paragraph for details.

can be analyzed in the *time* domain (voltage y-axis, time x-axis), the way clinicians are used to viewing them, or in the *frequency* domain (power y-axis, frequency x-axis). We will talk further about frequency mapping later (see Section 3.1.7), but for now suffice it to say that frequency analysis can reveal things we are blind to in time domain electrograms. Thus, when the investigators demonstrate that the rate of rotors correlates with the dominant frequency of the EKG, it implies that the rotors are the *cause* of the dominant frequency of the EKG.

In an optical mapping study of AF (Langendorff-perfused sheep hearts with acetylcholine), rotors were identified as phase singularities on the optical maps. These *driver sites were spatially stable* [42].

Analysis of bipolar electrograms was performed because intracardiac electrograms give location-specific information not provided by the body surface EKG. Electrograms revealed not only that the dominant frequency of the electrogram correlated with the frequency of the optically observed rotors, but also that the dominant frequency of the electrogram varied from location to location. High dominant frequency sites spatially correlated with phase singularities/ rotor sites [42], suggesting that

drivers can be located via electrogram recordings.

Zou et al., in Nattel's group, studied the role of substrate size on duration of fibrillation (i.e. the mass hypothesis). They used a mathematical model of AF with realistic action potentials and conduction properties. They induced AF in the presence of various concentrations and distributions of acetylcholine. What they found was interesting: "For large mean [ACh], single primary rotors anchored in low-[ACh] zones maintained activity *and substrate dimensions were not critical*. At lower mean [ACh], extensive spiral wave meander prevented the emergence of single stable rotors … when substrate size permitted a sufficiently large number of simultaneous longer-lasting rotors … extinction of all was unlikely" (emphasis added) [43].

This demonstrates the important point that with focal (spatially stable) drivers, the mass hypothesis shouldn't apply. Conversely, when one observes a *dependence of AF duration on tissue dimensions*, it implies a role for moving circuits.

Micro-reentry

There has been a theme in studies of AF mechanisms: we either have robust detailed data in a non-human experimental model (e.g. optical mapping, histology),[42] or limited data in humans (electrograms of varied resolution and distribution). These approaches to the study of fibrillation have often led to discrepant conclusions regarding the mechanisms that drive AF. This has raised the question of whether the discrepancies are due to differences in the models or in the adequacy of the data acquired. Fedorov's group has introduced some extremely valuable data into this landscape: tremendously robust data – gadolinium-enhanced magnetic resonance imaging (MRI), histology, and simultaneous endocardial, epicardial, and transmural panoramic optical mapping – *in explanted human hearts*. Their results, as we shall discuss, provide an additional interesting wrinkle: they indicate that the *apparent* mechanism of fibrillation can vary depending upon the heart surface mapped (endocardial versus epicardial).

Using a perfused, explanted, human lateral right atrial preparation, they correlated detailed anatomic data with transmural optical mapping data [44]. They were only able to induce sustained fibrillation after perfusing the heart with pinacidil, an IK_{ATP} channel opener, which shortens APD.[43] Under these conditions, sustained fibrillation was driven by structural micro-reentry. Importantly, the circuit was *transmural*, thus the complete circuit was not contained on either the epi- or endocardial surface. They demonstrated that the *perceived* mechanism of fibrillation varied depending upon the surface mapped; activation revealed a complete or incomplete reentrant circuit viewed from the endocardium, and appeared as a complete or incomplete reentrant circuit or as stable or unstable focal activation (breakthroughs) when viewed from the epicardial surface (Figure 37). Frequency analysis indicated spatiotemporal stability and electrogram dominant frequency matched the frequency of the micro-reentry.

Meticulous analysis revealed that reentry depended upon the architecture of the atrium. Variation in tissue thickness, interstitial fibrosis, and divergent endo- versus epicardial fiber orientation contributed to circuit formation [44]. The physiological impact of these architectural features appeared to be the creation of slowed conduction (endo- to epicardial conduction delay was seen

---

[42] And in computational studies, complete information.

[43] Epicardial APD 80 was decreased from 282.9 ± 47 to 158.7 ± 61; and endocardial APD 80 from 284.9 ± 45 to 165.3 ± 64 (500 ms pace cycle length).

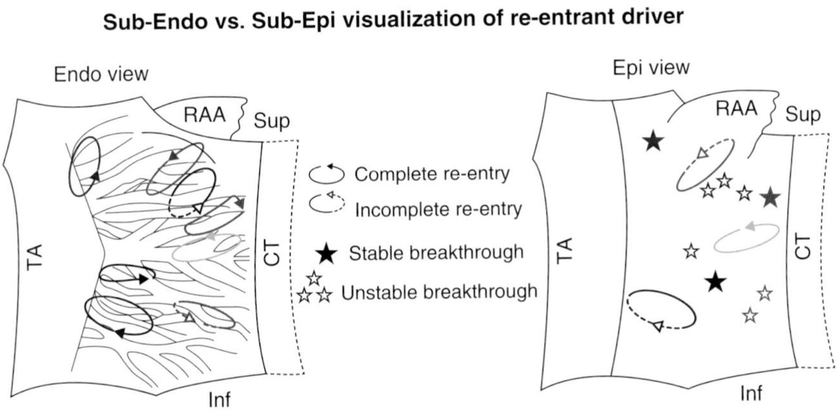

Sub-Endo vs. Sub-Epi visualization of re-entrant driver

Figure 37 **Appearance of driver varies depending upon which surface of the atrium is mapped.** (Left) Endocardial view, (right) epicardial view. Drivers appeared as either complete or incomplete circuits, stable breakthrough, or unstable breakthrough (legend). CT, crista terminalis; Inf, inferior vena cava; RAA, right atrial appendage; Sup, superior vena cava; TA, tricuspid annulus. *Source*: Reproduced with permission from [44].

to increase with wall thickness) and partial protection/insulation[44] resulting from endomysial fibrosis [44].

In a subsequent study, the same group performed similar detailed analyses of fibrillation in a *whole intact human bi-atrial preparation*. They once again found structural micro-reentry driving AF. The investigators examined the macro- and microscopic anatomic features with gadolinium-enhanced MRI and histology. Wall thickness varied throughout the atria: a greater percentage of the tissue in driver regions had a thickness of 20–30% of the maximal tissue thickness. They also examined the extent of fibrosis. In driver regions, a greater percentage of the tissue had 20–30% fibrosis [45]. Driver regions also tended to have a greater degree of misalignment of fiber orientation between endo- and epicardial layers. In this same study the investigators performed computational modeling. The same micro-reentrant driver of fibrillation was induced, but only when fibrosis and anisotropy were incorporated into the model [45].

Endocardial/epicardial discontinuities and atrial fibrillation

These were not the first studies to highlight the presence and importance

---

[44] Fibrosis provided electrical separation of portions of the circuit from the surrounding atrium; this, as we shall discuss, reduces the ability of external waves to terminate or de-anchor micro-reentry.

of dissociation between the endo- and epicardial surfaces of the heart. In 1993, Schuessler et al. performed simultaneous recording of the endo- and epicardial surfaces of the canine atria in an excised perfused/super-fused tissue preparation. They found that there could be endo/epi dissociation where there were trabeculae underlying the epicardium or in thin regions where there was significant change in fiber orientation across the atrial wall (Figure 38) [46]. After addition of acetylcholine, they were able to induce transmural reentry.

Allessie and Schotten's group in Maastricht have studied endo/epi dissociation in depth as well. They point out that as remodeling occurs, there is a progressive loss of transmural electrical continuity [47]. They suggest that under normal conditions the epicardium acts to coordinate propagation in otherwise disconnected pectinate bundles (Figure 39). With loss of the smoothing effect of this epicardial "bridge," pectinate bundles are activated dyssynchronously (Figure 39) [48].

Allessie performed epicardial mapping[45] in 24 patients with long-standing persistent AF and compared these with 25 patients with sinus rhythm in whom AF was induced. They analyzed 4403 maps of AF. *In no case* did they observe stable foci or rotors. Instead, they saw many narrow wavelets separated by lines of shifting functional block (Figure 40) [49]. They observed very large numbers of focal discharges on both surfaces of the heart which, based on the presence of R waves, they attributed to breakthrough of activation from the opposite surface (Figure 41) [50].[46] The number of breakthroughs was markedly increased during persistent AF (as compared with induced AF; Figure 42) [50]. In a follow-up study, they simultaneously mapped the endo- and epicardial surfaces of the right atrium in 10 AF patients (3 paroxysmal, 4 persistent, and 3 longstanding persistent). They found asynchronous transmural activation (which they defined as >15 ms difference in activation time on opposite surfaces), which was seen in 0.9–55.9% of recording sites, with equal distribution on the endo- and epicardial surfaces [51]. Of 1199 focal fibrillation waves, 65% were demonstrated to be breakthroughs based upon the

---

[45] 244 electrodes, 0.3 mm, interelectrode spacing 2.25 mm.

---

[46] When a wave of excitation propagates *only* away from a unipolar electrode (not toward and then away), the electrogram is negative and then positive (Q wave). If the wave first approaches the electrode (e.g. from the opposite surface of the heart), there is first a positive deflection (R wave) followed by a negative deflection (hence an rS pattern).

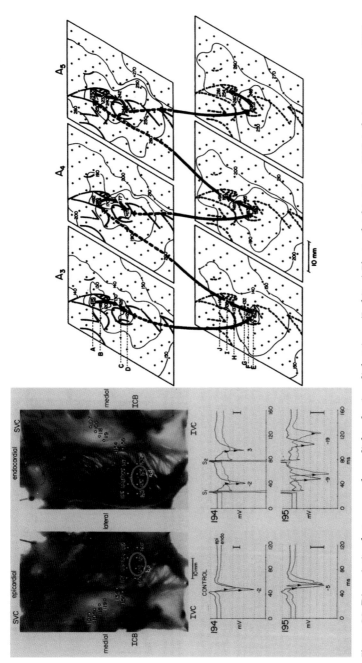

Figure 38 Dissociation between endocardial and epicardial atrium. (Left/top) Photo of right atrium. IVC, inferior vena cava; SVC, superior vena cava. (Left/bottom) Electrograms from epicardium (top tracing) and endocardium (bottom tracing) at the sites marked with a red circle, showing delayed conduction. (Right) Path of propagation for transmural reentry. *Source:* Reproduced with permission from [46].

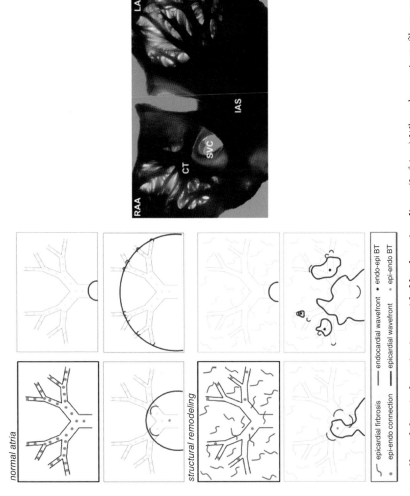

Figure 39 **Homogenizing effect of electrical continuity provided by the epicardium.** (Left/top) When the pectinate fibers are well connected to the overlying epicardium, propagation in the pectinates is synchronized. (Bottom) When the epicardium is electrically discontinuous with the pectinates, propagation is no longer synchronized. (Right) Photo of trans-illuminated atrium illustrating pectinate fibers. BT, breakthrough; CT, crista terminalis; IAS, interatrial septum; LAA, left atrial appendage; RAA, right atrial appendage; SVC, superior vena cava. *Source:* Reproduced with permission from [47].

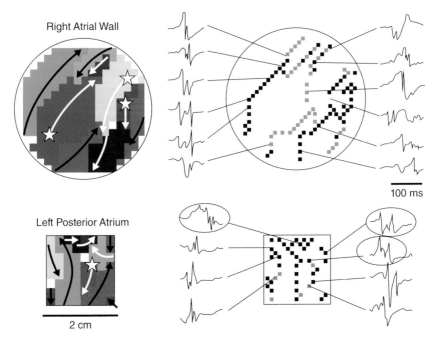

Figure 40 **Mapping of human atrial fibrillation**. Mapping revealed multiple narrow wave fronts and focal activations. Waves were reconstructed from meticulous analysis of electrograms. *Source*: Reproduced with permission from [49].

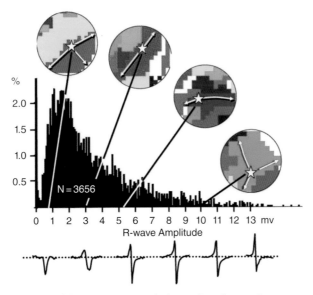

Figure 41 **Histogram of electrogram morphologies based upon R wave amplitude**. Focal activation patterns were interpreted as either de novo activations or transmural breakthrough sites based upon the presence or absence of R waves. The presence of an R wave was interpreted to mean that the wave approached from the opposite side of the atrial wall. *Source*: Reproduced with permission from [50].

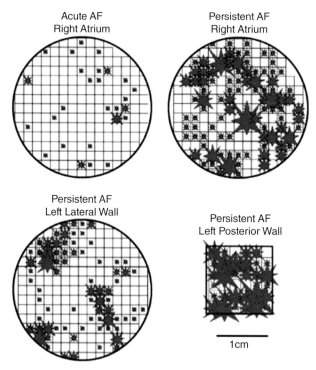

Figure 42 Distribution of wave breakthrough sites. Epicardial activation mapping during atrial fibrillation (AF) in humans revealed multiple breakthroughs; the number increased markedly in persistent (top right and bottom) compared with paroxysmal AF (top left). *Source*: Reproduced with permission from [50].

presence of a fibrillation wave on the opposite wall within 4 mm and 15 ms before the origin of the focal wave.

Anchoring of moving circuits

The capacity of meandering rotors (functional reentry) to anchor to an anatomic obstacle has been well established. In an elegant and simple series of experiments, the group from Cedars-Sanai examined the ability of meandering rotors to attach to holes of various sizes "punched" into superfused sheets of canine right atrial tissue, superfused with acetylcholine (Figure 43) [27]. They created holes (2–10 mm diameter) in the center of rectangular tissue (3.8×3.2 cm). Mapping was performed with 509 bipolar electrodes.[47] Rotors were induced with premature stimuli. In the absence of a hole, rotors meandered until they

---

[47] 0.4 mm, interbipolar spacing 0.5 mm, site spacing 1.6 mm.

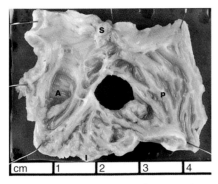

Figure 43 Structural obstacle in atrial tissue. A series of experiments were performed on excised and perfused atrial tissue with structural holes of varied size. Functional reentry was induced with programmed stimulation. Activation was mapped with multi-site simultaneous electrogram recordings. A, appendage; I, inferior; p, pectinate; S, superior. *Source*: Reproduced with permission from [27].

collided with a tissue boundary and were annihilated (or were induced to do so by a premature stimulus). Rotors did not anchor to holes of 2–4 mm (n = 6). The wave could propagate around the hole, but would "lift off," such that the wave tip was not in constant contact with the edge of the hole (Figure 44). The cells at the edge of the hole (where lift-off occurred) were excitable (and not refractory), as evidenced by intracellular micro-electrode recordings. The authors propose an interesting explanation for the lack of complete anchoring to small holes. At the edge of a small hole (which has a tighter curvature than a larger hole) there is a greater sink. This causes source-sink mismatch and failure to excite these cells even though they are not refractory (Figure 45) [27]. With 6 mm, 8 mm (n = 8 each), and 10 mm (n = 6) holes, rotors became anchored, converting functional into structural reentry and polymorphic electrograms (recorded during meander) into monomorphic, periodic electrograms. The cycle length of reentry was reduced upon anchoring and correlated with the circumference of the hole.

In a follow-up study, the same group looked at the role of pectinate muscles in atrial tachycardia and fibrillation. Once again they used an isolated superfused canine right atrial preparation. During regular pacing (cycle length 300 ms) there was no evidence of conduction block and no impact of pectinate bundles on conduction velocity [2]. In the absence of acetylcholine, fewer than 10 beats of reentry could be induced with premature stimuli. During acetylcholine perfusion, the refractory period was reduced (117 ± 17 ms vs. 66 ± 19 ms) and 40 episodes of reentry were induced; 28 of these episodes were stationary reentry (mean cycle length 116 ± 22 ms), 20 of which were spiral wave reentry and 8 were structural reentry using a pectinate muscle "bridge."[48] In 12 episodes there was meandering functional reentry

---

[48] A pectinate muscle bridge exists when the pectinate is attached to the atrial epicardium at both ends but not in the middle.

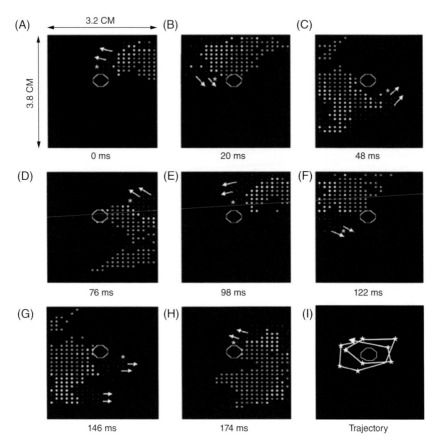

Figure 44 Propagation around a 4 mm diameter hole. A functional reentrant circuit propagated around obstacles, but when holes were too small rotors could not remain anchored to the edge of the obstacle. (Asterisk indicates wave tip: note where it is separated from the edge of the hole – all panels except H.) Cells at the edge were excitable (as demonstrated by intracellular action potential recordings), suggesting source-sink mismatch as the mechanism of de-anchoring. *Source*: Reproduced with permission from [27].

(mean cycle length 68 ± 11 ms). During structural reentry, which was slower, conduction was 1 : 1 to the remainder of the tissue, producing atrial tachycardia, whereas during faster, functional reentry, propagation was irregular, producing fibrillation. The investigators postulated that at the site where the relatively thin atrial epicardium joins the thick pectinate muscle, source-sink mismatch produced unidirectional conduction block. At

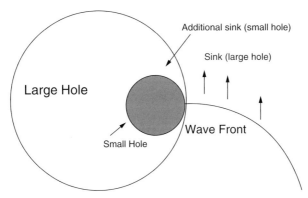

Figure 45 Postulated mechanism of de-anchoring from small holes. When hole size is too small, the curvature at the edge of the hole was postulated to be too steep, producing source-sink mismatch and failure of conduction. A represents incrementally increased sink area due to smaller-radius hole. *Source*: Reproduced with permission from [27].

slower pace cycle lengths (in the absence of premature stimulation), APD is longer (due to restitution), thus the source current is larger and propagation succeeds at the atrial pectinate muscle junction. During premature stimuli, APD, upstroke velocity, and amplitude are reduced, resulting in source-sink mismatch and block [2].

The interaction between fibrillation and atrial architecture was studied in a sheep model of heart failure.[49] Histological examination revealed that the sheep developed increased fibrosis (compared with baseline). In heart failure, patches were more numerous, larger, and more peripherally located (adjacent to the pulmonary

vein ostia) [52]. Examination of atrial activation in the posterior left atrial wall revealed predominantly high-frequency breakthroughs in both control and heart failure, but in the heart failure group these tended to be more peripheral, at the vein ostia. Once again, these studies demonstrate the impact of atrial architecture on the distribution of waves during fibrillation.

It is clear that the atria are capable of complex activation patterns. Stationary or meandering rotors can be initiated depending upon the excitability and wave length of the tissue. Meandering rotors can anchor to various anatomic features, converting a rotor into a functional reentrant circuit. Finally, structural circuits, partially protected by fibrosis, can sustain micro-reentry at rates fast

---

[49] Ventricular pacing (220 bpm for six to seven weeks) induced heart failure.

enough to cause fibrillatory conduction. It is not surprising that with the range of atrial anatomy and the heterogeneity of electrophysiological properties (within atria and between patients), these varying types of AF drivers exist and co-exist [53].

Fibrillatory conduction or multi-wavelet reentry?

Since AF research began, there has been debate over the mechanism(s) responsible for its perpetuation. These arguments have largely centered around two particular mechanisms: focal drivers with fibrillatory conduction and multi-wavelet reentry. Most (but certainly not all) investigators either explicitly state or at least imply that the two are mutually exclusive. In at least one case (data which indicated that AF, in a particular canine model, was due to focal drivers with fibrillatory conduction), it was argued that focal drivers with fibrillatory conduction must be the mechanism of AF in *all cases*.[50] As we've already reviewed, it is clear that atrial fibrillation can result from several different mechanisms. The mechanism in any particular case

depends upon that tissue's physiology. Thus, if anything, the debate could be: Which of the known potential mechanisms for AF is *the* mechanism in humans? Because different mechanisms result from different tissue properties, another way to ask this question would be: What is the underlying tissue physiology in humans? But it is overwhelmingly likely that humans have a wide range of physiologies, from patient to patient, time to time, and location to location. In fact, multiple mechanisms can co-exist at the same time in the same patient; there is no reason to believe that these are mutually exclusive physiological behaviors.

Thus far we've been discussing *drivers*: multi-wavelet reentry, focal rotors, and micro-reentry. Regardless of driver type, *fibrillation* is only present if the driver results in changing activation patterns. For multi-wavelet reentry, the driver itself has changing activation patterns, due to the nature of spatially dynamic functional circuits. In the case of focal rotors, or micro-reentry, whether we classify the rhythm as AF or atrial tachycardia depends *not* upon the type of driver; rather, it depends upon how waves emanating from the driver *propagate*: 1 : 1 equals atrial tachycardia, shifting block equals fibrillation. When conduction through the atria is *not* 1 : 1 it is described as *fibrillatory*

---

[50] It is a logical fallacy to state that the proof of the existence of one thing must mean the proof of the lack of existence of another.

conduction. In this part of our story I'd like to dig deeper into fibrillatory conduction itself.

Is fibrillatory conduction active or passive?

Jalife's group did an interesting study of fibrillatory conduction. In a Langendorff-perfused sheep model of AF,[51] they studied fibrillatory conduction using optical and phase mapping. Phase maps allowed them to identify phase singularities and then determine the relationships between wave fronts and phase singularities. Wave breaks produced phase singularities, which formed frequently (~70/400 ms recording). Wave break actually creates two phase singularities (at both broken ends). Depending upon the distance between the two there could be double-loop (or "figure-of-eight") reentry (Figure 46). When the phase singularities were too close together (<~4 mm), there was source-sink mismatch as the wave passed between the phase singularities and both rotors terminated [54] (Figure 47).[52] In the majority of instances, phase singularities were very short lived (mean duration 19.5 ± 18.3 ms), lasting less than one rotation. Phase singularities that fail to complete a single rotation are appropriately referred to as fibrillatory conduction, in that they cannot self-sustain (there is no reentry) and hence are completely dependent upon their driver.[53] On the other hand, when phase singularities were more than 4 mm apart, two counter-rotating waves were produced, which were able to sustain themselves. These could also interact with *other* waves, inducing further wave break, annihilation, or meander. Thus, one can see how a focal driver could act to "stoke" multi-wavelet reentry by inducing the formation of functional reentrant circuits as well as inducing meander of these circuits.

The investigators sought to directly test the hypothesis that these wavelets were *not maintaining fibrillation*. To this end, they compared the number of waves entering their field of view with the number of waves leaving the field. The logic was that if the region was driving fibrillation, it would emit more waves than it received. The mean number of waves entering was greater than those leaving (15.7 ± 1.6 vs. 9.7 ± 1.5 [p < 0.01]) [54]. This result suggested to the investigators that the region *observed* was not

---

[51] Using perfusion with acetyl choline 0.1–0.5 μM.

[52] This is directly analogous to a narrow accessory pathway inserting into much broader ventricular tissue.

---

[53] Whatever generated the wave that "broke."

(A)   (B)

(C)   (D)

(E)   (F)

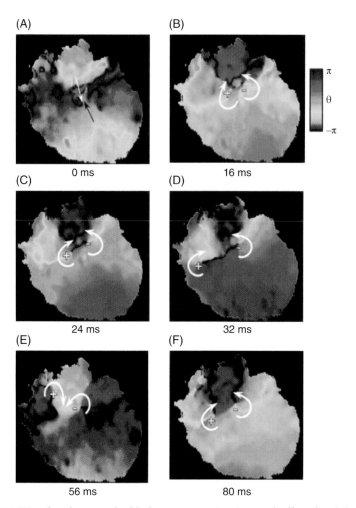

Figure 46 Wave break causes double-loop reentry. In a Langendorff-perfused sheep model of atrial fibrillation, wave break (A) produced two counter-rotating waves (B–F). *Source*: Reproduced with permission from [54].

driving fibrillation. They proposed that this supports the notion of a focal rotor driving passive fibrillatory conduction rather than multi-wavelet reentry. Taken in isolation, one might argue that it doesn't specifically require that it be rotors that drove fibrillation in this case. It could simply be that the driver, regardless of mechanism, arose in a location outside the observed region; i.e. it could be seen with multi-wavelet

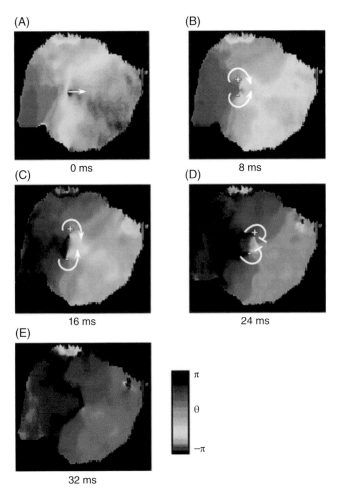

Figure 47 Closely spaced rotor cores terminate. When phase singularities were too closely spaced, source-sink mismatch (as the wave tried to exit from between the cores) resulted in block and termination. (A) Wave front (green) propagating left to right. (B) Wave break at refractory tissue (red) causes counter-rotating rotors. (C) Propagation occurs around the outside of the phase singularities, but (D) the wave cannot emerge from between the phase singularities due to source-sink mismatch. (E) Termination of rotors. *Source*: Reproduced with permission from [54].

reentry in which circuit density is concentrated in a region (or regions) outside of the one they observed. However, when you combine the ratio of waves entering/leaving with their other work, in which they've demonstrated spatiotemporal regularity [41], it suggests that the driver of fibrillation in these studies is *regular* (e.g. a focal rotor).[54]

Can fibrillatory conduction be active?

It is generally implied that fibrillatory conduction is always a passive, driven behavior. In fact, the premise of the ablation strategy – find the driver and ablate it – depends upon the assumption that, without the driver, fibrillatory conduction (and hence fibrillation) will cease. Let's consider whether that assumption is *necessarily* valid.

One way to approach this question is to ask how fibrillatory conduction *could be* self-sustaining (i.e. independent of a driver). *If* it were to sustain itself, it would entail ongoing propagation (that lasts longer than the time required for a wave to conduct across a tissue of finite extent). This requires reexcitation of cells that have already been excited, which requires circuits and reentry. How would this be different from multi-wavelet reentry? It wouldn't.

In both fibrillatory conduction and multi-wavelet reentry, rapid rates and heterogeneous refractoriness produce variable conduction [55–57].

We hypothesized that fibrillatory conduction and multi-wavelet reentry differ only in the extent to which wave break produces functional reentrant circuits and the capacity of a particular tissue to sustain these circuits. As such, fibrillatory conduction and multi-wavelet reentry represent two points along a continuum. In atria with minimal capacity to support functional reentry, changing propagation is passive and dependent upon the presence of drivers (see earlier discussion). In tissues with a greater ability to sustain functional reentry, variable conduction is self-sustaining, perpetuating even in the absence of drivers.

We used a computational model to test whether fibrillatory conduction would perpetuate in the absence of a driver.[55] We created 2D sheets of tissue (8×8 cm) with a structural micro-reentrant driver at the center. In the tissue surrounding the focal driver, we varied the wave length by varying APD (50–200 ms in 5 ms increments, with ±10 ms of random variation). Once fibrillatory conduction was present, structural reentry was eliminated by ablation of the entire central driver. The duration of fibrillation following driver elimination was measured (up to 10 000 seconds).

---

[54] One would not expect that multi-wavelet reentry would generate regular, periodic activity.

[55] Note: This study has not yet been published, and hence is not peer-reviewed.

Episode durations were compared with predictions based upon the fibrillogenicity index.

The focal driver produced either fibrillatory conduction or organized propagation (i.e. "atrial" tachycardia), depending upon driver rate relative to the surrounding tissue's refractoriness. Fibrillatory conduction resulted when driver cycle length fell between the longest and shortest refractory periods of the surrounding cells. Fibrillatory conduction **duration,** *after driver elimination*, increased with decreasing APD and was well predicted by the fibrillogenicity index (Figures 48 and 49C).[56] For APDs between 90 and 110 ms, there was 2 : 1 conduction with organized propagation (i.e. no fibrillatory conduction). Under these conditions, quiescence immediately followed driver elimination.[57]

These data demonstrate that fibrillatory conduction can be sustained in the absence of a driver. This is an important consideration when contemplating ablation of AF in the presence of focal drivers: *focal driver elimination is necessary but may not be sufficient.*[58]

These data have another significant implication: *focal drivers and multi-wavelet reentry can coexist.* This raises an important question: Can the two driver types influence one another, and if so, how? To examine this question, we did another series of computational studies.[59] We used the same tissue set-up described above (a central micro-reentrant circuit surrounded by tissue with varied capacity to sustain multi-wavelet reentry). We sought to determine (i) the dynamics of micro-reentry as a function of varying vulnerability to external waves and (ii) the impact that the presence of the structural circuit had on the overall duration of fibrillation (i.e. irregular activation due to either micro-reentry, multi-wavelet reentry, or both).

---

[56] I.e. as the wave length of the tissue was reduced, its capacity to sustain functional reentrant circuits increased and "fibrillatory conduction" was in fact multi-wavelet reentry.

[57] This, too, makes the point that for *conduction* to be self-sustaining, it must propagate in reentrant loops. During 1 : 1 organized conduction, there is no wave break and no circuits, hence waves are all doomed to annihilation at the tissue borders.

[58] The term "driver" is often used to mean *focal* driver, as if to say that multi-wavelet reentry is not a driver. I prefer to say that *whatever* is responsible for perpetuating AF is a driver; thus drivers can be focal or more diffuse. Here too, I'd like to clarify: multi-wavelet reentry need not be a uniformly distributed driver. As we've already seen, short wave length regions can have a higher circuit core density than lower wave length regions.

[59] This study is not yet published.

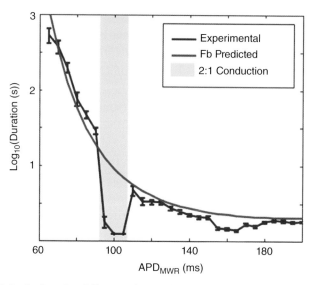

Figure 48 Episode duration following driver elimination. The duration of fibrillation following ablation of a micro-reentrant driver (blue line) was predicted by the fibrillogenicity (Fb) index (pink line). Note that when micro-reentry was propagated 2 : 1 (i.e. no fibrillatory conduction; gray bar), quiescence immediately followed driver elimination. (Error bars indicate standard error of the mean.) APD, action potential duration; MWR, multiple wavelet re-entry.

Dynamics of structural micro-reentry in the presence of multi-wavelet reentry

In the study just described, we examined propagation around the micro-reentrant circuit *during* multi-wavelet reentry/fibrillatory conduction. External waves can interact with structural reentry (entrainment, anti-tachycardia pacing) and with the structural reentrant circuit itself (unidirectional block and induction of reentry). We therefore tested the hypothesis that in the presence of an ongoing supply of waves (multi-wavelet reentry/fibrillatory conduction), reentry in a structural circuit would be serially induced and terminated, and that the cadence of induction/termination would be dependent upon the ability of waves to *reach* and penetrate the structural circuit. We varied the degree of continuity between the structural circuit and the surrounding tissue, and the relative rates of structural and multi-wavelet reentry.

Activation within the structural circuit alternated between **reentry** (Figure 49B-1) (induced by unidirectional block of an entering wave) and

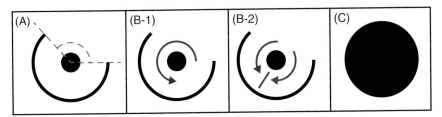

Figure 49 Micro-reentrant circuit. (A) We created a circuit for structural reentry in the center of a two-dimensional sheet of simulated tissue. The circuit had a central obstacle partially surrounded by a semi-circle of scar. Activation within the circuit could be reentry (B-1), or bidirectional conduction and mutual annihilation at the far side of the circuit (B-2). The driver was eliminated by ablating the entire circuit (C).

passive bidirectional activation following reentry termination via bidirectional block (Figure 49B-2), with wave collision opposite from the wave entry site. The percentage of time for which there was reentry in the structural circuit varied with (i) the relative rate *of the multi-wavelet reentry* and (ii) the degree of circuit protection (continuity with the surrounding tissue; Figure 49A). A greater percentage of time was spent in structural reentry, as the rate of multi-wavelet reentry increased from slower than to equal to the rate of structural reentry (Figure 50A). As multi-wavelet reentry rate increased further (greater than the rate of structural reentry), the structural circuit was able to maintain reentry less and less often. The extent of circuit protection (decreasing exposure of the circuit to the surrounding tissue) markedly increased the stability of structural reentry (Figure 50B).

Initiation and termination of structural reentry require access of waves to the structural circuit. As APD decreases (in the tissue surrounding the structural circuit), multi-wavelet reentry rate increases. Thus, the number of waves, and therefore interactions with the structural circuit, increase as well. This leads to a corresponding decrease in the percentage of time for which there is stable reentry around the structural circuit; the circuit is under constant bombardment by incoming waves. Likewise, increasing circuit exposure allows fibrillatory waves to approach from more directions,[60] causing a decrease in the likelihood of stable wave anchoring. When multi-wavelet and structural reentry rates are the same, the percentage of time during which waves are anchored peaks (Figure 50A).

---

[60] And the excitable gap is exposed more of the time.

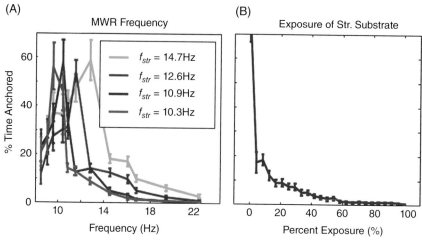

Figure 50 Percentage of time there was reentry in the micro-reentrant circuit. (A) Reentry was serially induced and terminated in the presence of fibrillatory conduction. The amount of time spent with reentry around the circuit varied with the relative frequencies of the structural reentry vs. average frequency of fibrillatory conduction (fibrillatory rates inset). (B) Percentage of time with structural reentry also varied with the amount of circuit protection. Note that in the absence of protection, the micro-reentrant circuit could not support reentry. MWR, multiple wavelet re-entry.

The focal driver and multi-wavelet reentry are unable to entrain one another, so, once initiated, structural reentry continues largely unmolested. Counter-intuitively, long APD (slower multi-wavelet reentry) also causes a drop in the percentage of time spent in structural reentry. In this case, waves emitted by the relatively faster structural reentry collide with refractory tissue directly adjacent to the structural circuit. This leads to wave break in the immediate vicinity of the circuit. The waves produced are well positioned to penetrate the circuit and interrupt reentry.

Impact of a structural reentrant circuit on the average duration of multi-wavelet reentry

Having demonstrated that multi-wavelet reentry can interact with a structural reentrant circuit, we examined whether *the presence of a structural circuit* would increase, decrease, or not alter the average duration of fibrillation.

We initiated 500 episodes of multi-wavelet reentry (100 Hz burst pacing) and measured the time to spontaneous termination, in the presence and absence of a micro-reentrant circuit. In order to distinguish the role of altered tissue area from the role of the presence or absence of structural reentry, we tested both the absence of a circuit (thus more surface area for multi-wavelet reentry) and an ablated circuit (reduced surface area).

There was no difference in fibrillation duration in the absence of a circuit (no obstacles; Figure 51A) or following circuit ablation (Figure 51B). Interestingly, the presence of a structural circuit (Figure 51C) only increased the duration of fibrillation when the rate of structural reentry was greater than that of multi-wavelet reentry (Figure 51D). Thus, for tissues with long APD (hence a reduced ability to maintain multi-wavelet reentry), the mere presence of a structural circuit increased the duration of fibrillation. In this setting, structural reentry provides a source for new wave formation when multi-wavelet reentry would otherwise terminate spontaneously.

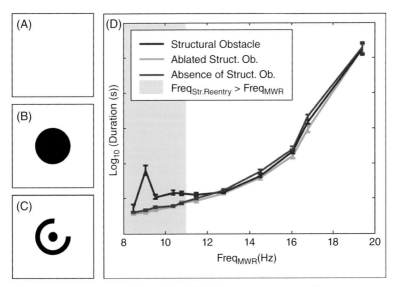

Figure 51 Duration of fibrillation with and without the presence of a micro-reentrant circuit. Duration of fibrillation was unchanged whether the circuit was absent (A and red line in D) or ablated (B and green line in D). In the presence of a micro-reentrant circuit (C and blue line in D), duration only increased when the frequency of micro-reentry was greater than that of fibrillatory conduction (gray bar, D). MWR, multiple wavelet re-entry.

Location of atrial fibrillation drivers

We've been discussing *what* drives AF. For an electrophysiologist interested in *fixing* fibrillation, knowledge of its mechanism is necessary, but *not sufficient*. We must also know *where* AF drivers are located. Because the atria are complex heterogeneous structures, fibrillation is not spatially homogeneous: there are gradients in physiology, frequency, and drivers of activation [2, 52, 58–67].

Regional gradients

Demonstrations of regional gradients during fibrillation abound, and here are a few examples.

Warren et al. demonstrated that there was a steep regional gradient of activation frequency during VF (in optical mapping of guinea pig heart), and that the gradient corresponded to a gradient in the amount of I_{K1} current (and its corresponding mRNA) [68]. The fastest site was a focal rotor driving VF; when I_{K1} current was blocked (with barium), APD was increased, rotation rate decreased, and VF terminated [68].

Regional gradients of ion channels and hence action potentials are present in human atria as well. Voigt et al. examined protein expression and current density in the right and left atria of patients with sinus rhythm and AF [69]. Baseline current was double in chronic AF patients compared with sinus (but there were no right to left current gradients). In patients with paroxysmal AF, there was around twofold greater I_{K1} and IK_{Ach} in the left versus the right atrium.

Regional gradients in *frequency* have been repeatedly demonstrated in patients with AF. In an epicardial atrial mapping study performed in 10 patients undergoing cardiac surgery, transient rotational drivers were identified (by multi-site simultaneous activation mapping) and the shortest cycle length (78 ± 4 ms) "consistently co-locate[d] to the core of rotation" [70].

In a study that almost fulfills Koch's postulates, Campbell et al. manipulated the amount of I_{Kr} expressed in cultures of rat neonatal ventricular myocytes, and examined the impact on spatial dispersion of APD, rotor localization, and frequency [71]. In 64 different monolayers, rotors were found in the high I_{Kr} region[61] 57.8% of the time, at the border between high and low I_{Kr} regions 18.8% of the time, and in the low I_{Kr} region 23.4% of the time ($P < 0.0001$) [71]. They also found that when the rotor was in the area with short APD there was

---

[61] Short APD.

wave break and fibrillatory conduction into the long APD region, but when the rotor was in the long APD region there was uniform 1 : 1 conduction (i.e. tachycardia, not fibrillation).

Which driver type and where?

The physiology we've been discussing tells us that there can be several different types of reentrant drivers of AF. Which type depends upon local electrophysiology (e.g. wave length, excitability, and hence meander) as well as tissue architecture (e.g. partially protected structural micro-reentrant circuits and anchoring). But electrophysiological properties and architecture vary across the atria. How does all the physiology play out to determine what happens where?

Why are fast sites *fast*?

There are consistently faster sites and slower sites[62] [58–60, 72, 73]. Fast sites are fast because… they can be (because of their refractory period).

This sounds flip, but it is not just obvious, it is explanatory. Remember, we are talking about fibrillation; if we weren't, all locations would (by definition) be going at the same rate. In fibrillation, there are different rates because some areas cannot follow others in 1 : 1 fashion. So, is it necessarily the regions that have the shortest refractory periods that tend to go the fastest? Is it not possible to have a site that produces waves at a rate faster than some of its immediate neighbors but nonetheless there are remote regions, with a refractory period short enough to follow 1 : 1, but which aren't because some waves fail to reach them?[63] Sure, not all cells are excited as quickly as they can be [74].[64] A cell's refractory period limits how fast it can be excited (it can't be excited *faster* than its refractory period allows). But its actual activation rate is not determined by its refractory period; cells are only excited as often as waves reach them – *the rate is set by the driver, not the follower.*

---

[62] If one location was faster now, but a different location was faster later, and if over time it turned out that all locations had an equal likelihood of being faster (at some points in time), then there would be very little value in identifying (or even talking about) regional gradients. This, in fact, is a key to mapping: there is only value in mapping (as a guide to ablation) if what you identify *at the time of the map* is also true at times when you are not mapping.

---

[63] I.e. regions of long refractory period *intervening* between the driver and tissue capable of rapid excitation limit the rate of the *driven* cells.

[64] It has been demonstrated that there are regions with an excitable gap during fibrillation.

Impact of regional heterogeneity on the dynamics of atrial fibrillation drivers

So your refractory period doesn't determine how fast you go, it simply constrains how fast you *can* go. **Drivers** determine how fast you go (think sinus rhythm). Driver rates are determined by local tissue electrophysiology. In the roiling dynamics of fibrillation, we need not simply consider the physiology that determines driver rate, we also need to focus on the word "local" in the prior sentence. First, as we've seen, some drivers are *moving*, so location is changing. Second, drivers can be terminated by outside waves, and they only set rate *when they are "driving"* (i.e. once terminated they no longer determine local rate). So, in order to sort out "which driver type and where" we need to discuss *how* a driver's spatial stability has an impact on regional driver distribution and *how* interactions between drivers influence which drivers survive and which are terminated.

Tissue properties and spatial stability

Rotors with small cores are *faster and more stationary* than rotors with larger cores. This was examined in a model of stretch-induced fibrillation. Optical maps of Langendorff-perfused sheep hearts revealed that dominant frequency co-localized with areas of shortest APD [28]. Infusion of chloroquine (an I_{K1} blocker which slowed rotors) increased core size *and increased rotor susceptibility to termination* via *external waves* (Figure 52) [28]. In transgenic mouse hearts, upregulation of I_{K1} produced ventricular fibrillation driven by stable high-frequency rotors (37 Hz; phase singularity trajectory <1 mm). Chloroquine decreased rotor dominant frequency (to 22 Hz) and increased the distance that rotors moved (PS trajectory ~4 mm), causing meander into boundaries and termination [75]. In the Langendorff-perfused guinea pig heart, VF was driven by a rapid rotor in the left ventricle (LV; 25–30 Hz; Figure 53), with fibrillatory conduction to the slower right ventricle [RV] [76]. Associated computational modeling studies suggested that increased I_{K1} in the LV accelerated and stabilized rotors (Figure 54) [76]. In a tachy-pacing–induced sheep model of AF, APD decreased due to reduced I_{Ca} and I_{Na}, and increased I_{K1}. The authors used computational modeling to study the impact of these ion current changes on AF dynamics. As APD decreased, rotors slowed and drifted, eventually colliding with the tissue boundary, terminating fibrillation (Figure 55) [77].

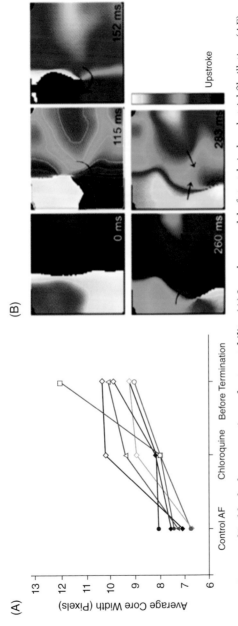

Figure 52 Impact of I_{K1} blockade on core size and rotor stability. (A) In a sheep model of stretch-induced atrial fibrillation (AF), blockade of I_{K1} with chloroquine increased core size (B) and increased rotor susceptibility to termination by external waves. *Source:* Reproduced with permission from [3].

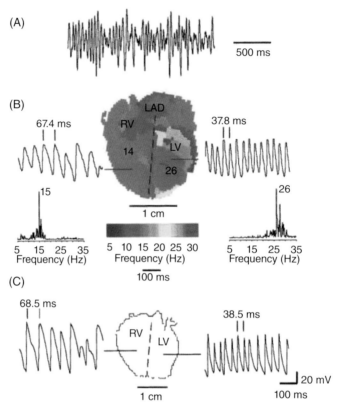

Figure 53 **In Langendorff-perfused guinea pig hearts, upregulation of I_{K1} caused rapid ventricular fibrillation driven from the left ventricle** (LV). (A) Electrocardiogram. (B) Dominant frequency derived from optical mapping. (C) Intracellular micro-electrode recordings correlate with dominant frequency maps. LAD, left anterior descending artery; RV, right ventricle. *Source*: Reproduced with permission from [76].

The cellular physiology of pulmonary veins and posterior left atrial cells was compared in canines. Pulmonary vein cells had a higher resting membrane potential, lower action potential amplitude, smaller maximum phase 0 upstroke velocity, and shorter APD. Sodium current density was similar in the vein and the LA, suggesting that reduced upstroke was due to resting depolarization and increased sodium channel inactivation in the pulmonary vein. Inward rectifier current density in the vein was lower than the atrium (likely resulting in the less negative resting

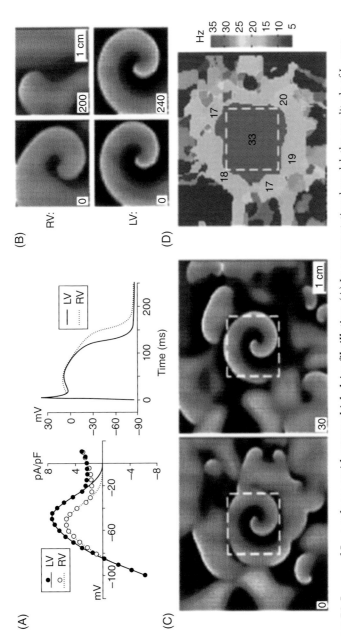

Figure 54 Increased I$_{K1}$ produces rapid rotors which drive fibrillation. (A) In a computational model, the amplitude of I$_{K1}$ was modified via alteration of rectification – increased current in left ventricle (LV) and decreased action potential duration. (B) Rotors were unstable in the presence of longer wave length. RV, right ventricle. (C, D) When there was a central patch with increased I$_{K1}$, a rapid stable central rotor drove slower fibrillatory conduction in the surrounding tissue. *Source:* Reproduced with permission from [76].

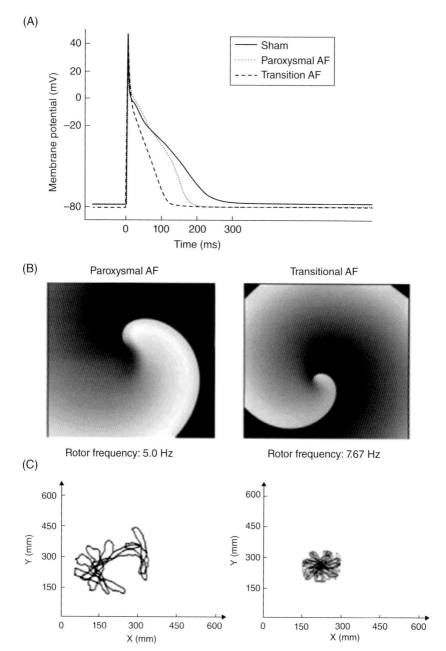

Figure 55 Action potential duration alters rotor stability. (A) In a computational model, action potential duration (APD) was altered to mimic normal, paroxysmal, and transition to persistent atrial fibrillation (AF) physiology. (B, C) Decreasing APD caused rotors to increase rate and decrease meander. *Source*: Reproduced with permission from [77].

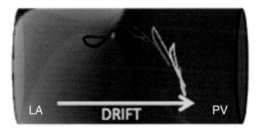

Figure 56 Rotor drift toward pulmonary vein. Computational modeling of a gradient in conductance of I_{K1} – larger in the left atrium (LA), smaller at the pulmonary vein (PV) – resulted in rotor drift from LA toward PV. *Source*: Modified with permission from [79].

membrane potential).[65] I_{Kr} and I_{Ks} were larger, while I_{to} and I_{Ca++L} were smaller in the vein [78]. Computational modeling of these ion channel changes resulted in meandering of rotors from the posterior LA to the ostium of the pulmonary vein (Figure 56) [79].

Cores in the setting of interactions with other waves

An otherwise stable rotor can be made to meander (and to collide with a boundary and annihilate itself) by interaction with other waves (Figures 57 and 58). In a study of isolated superfused canine atrial tissue, reentry was induced (programmed stimulation) and mapped (509 bipolar electrodes).[66] After 15

episodes of functional reentry were induced, in 13 of the 15 termination was induced when interaction between an external wave and the rotor caused meander and termination at the edge of the tissue. In 2 of the 15 an external wave of opposite direction from the rotation resulted in direct collision and annihilation [10]. Interactions between rotors and paced waves was studied in a computational model. Responses fell into three groups: rotor drift (Figure 57A), wave break of spiral arms with new rotor formation (Figure 57B), or no effect [80]. The result of the interaction depended upon stimulus timing, amplitude, and location relative to the rotor core. Pacing induced wave breaks at the cathode and the anode. Rotor drift resulted from interaction between the initial rotor and these pace-induced rotors. What appeared as drift was actually

---

[65] I_{K1} largely sets resting membrane potential.
[66] 0.4 mm diameter, 0.5 mm intrabipolar spacing, and 1.6 mm interbipolar spacing.

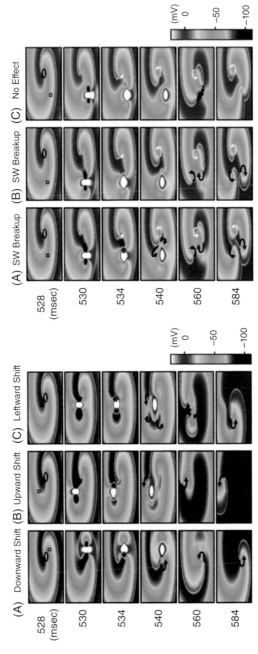

Figure 57 **Interactions between rotors and paced waves.** Computational modeling revealed that the impact of pacing on a rotor depended upon the spatial relationship between the rotor core and the site of pacing. (Left) When pacing was near to the core, there was a shift in the position of the rotor. (Right) When pacing was farther away, interaction between pacing and the rotor's spiral arm caused spiral wave (SW) break. *Source:* Reproduced with permission from [80].

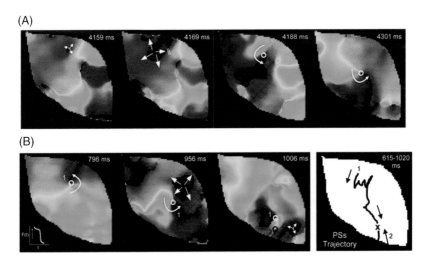

Figure 58 **Rotor drift and termination via interaction with an external wave**. (A) In a sheep model of stretch-induced fibrillation, focal firing induced rotors. (B) Further focal firing caused rotor drift and, often, annihilation. *Source*: Reproduced with permission from [81].

termination of the original rotor (due to collision with the counter-rotating paced wave) and "shift" was in fact to the location of the pace-induced rotor (Figure 57A) [80].

In a sheep, atrial stretch model of fibrillation, AF was maintained by focal firing (which resulted from triggered firing). When the heart was exposed to adrenergic stimulation, focal discharges caused wave break and rotor initiation (Figure 58). Once rotors were initiated, interaction with focal waves caused rotor drift and often boundary collision/termination. When these tissues were subsequently perfused with either ryanodine or caffeine,[67]

focal discharges were abolished and stable long-lasting rotors resulted [81].

Variable meander distance and rotor distribution

As described earlier, a circuit can meander because its wave front hits its own tail. Excitability and wave length determine whether cores will meander and how far. Can we simply ignore the details of physiology and predict where moving circuits will cluster based upon *regional differences in how far cores meander*? Perhaps. Imagine our drunk walkers (from Section 2.3.6.1.2). What would happen if they not only walked in random directions, but took different-size steps depending upon where they were? This (in very simplistic terms) describes the behavior of

---

[67] Which abolish intracellular calcium release–related triggered firing.

moving cores: regional variations in tissue wave length and excitability produce regional variations in meander distance. When cores are in an area of large movement, they will tend to move away from that area. When they (randomly) wind up in an area where movement is smaller, they will tend to settle there. Figure 59 shows the result of modeling a simplistic 2D random walk, with and without regions of smaller "step size." We programmed the 2D random walk model so that when a "core" hit a boundary, it was annihilated and a new core started at a random location on the tissue. By tracing the core's movement, we can see where it has been and how much time it has spent in each location. When there were no gradients in step size, cores were homogeneously distributed (Figure 59A), as is the case with circuit cores in homogeneous tissues. But when there was a short-step region, cores spent much more time in this area (Figure 59B and C). This behavior largely recapitulates our multi-wavelet

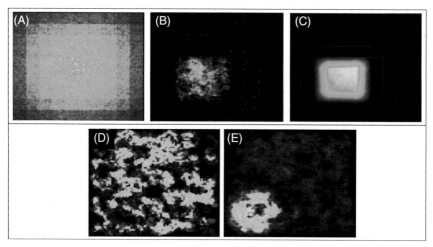

Figure 59 Regional gradients in core meander distance determine core distribution. (A) In a two-dimensional random walk, where step size is uniform, "walker density" is relatively homogeneous (note that there is lower density at the edges because the walker "annihilates" when it reaches the edge). (B) When there is a region with smaller step size, "walker density" is highest in this region. (C) The "walker gradient" is higher when the simulation is run for longer. The distribution of circuit cores displays the same behavior. (D) With homogeneous tissue properties, circuit core density is homogeneously distributed. (E) When there is a short wave length patch, circuit core density is highest in the patch. *Source*: (A–C) Reproduced with permission from Visible Electrophysiology LLC. (D, E) Reproduced with permission from [82].

reentry modeling studies (which include the physiological complexities of wave behavior). Circuit core density was homogeneously distributed in the absence of a short wave length patch (Figure 59D), but when there was a region with shorter APD, circuit core density was higher there (Figure 59E).

Where are driver sites?

Circuits start at sites of wave break. As we just discussed, moving circuits tend to cluster where movement is minimal. Because circuit movement relates to wave length and excitability, the regions with the highest density of circuit cores in multi-wavelet reentry are determined by those tissue properties that modify wave length and excitability.

What about structural circuits? They don't move, so surely where they start *is* where they settle… right?

They start where the circuit is (i.e. micro-reentry) or where tissue architecture creates source-sink mismatch and wave break. But we will see that, even for structural circuits, the question isn't where they form but whether they *remain* there.[68] This, as we'll discuss, depends upon their interactions with other drivers. So, in order to bet-

ter understand "what types of drivers and where," we need to dig a little deeper into the principles that guide the interactions between drivers.

Principles of propagation: Driver interactions in fibrillation

We've talked about where *a* driver will end up, but what about when there are multiple drivers?

Excited cells fall into two categories: those that participate in actively driving waves, and those that passively follow. When there are multiple drivers, different cells follow different drivers. We can think of drivers as competing for *excitable* cells; drivers are the predators and followers are the prey. What determines the dynamics of this competition? The following reviews some of the basics of how waves interact with each other *in general*. This is the first step toward understanding how *drivers* interact with each other during fibrillation.

Waves and wave sources

During sinus rhythm the atria are driven by the sinus node. However, the atrial wave breaks into two waves, one traversing the HPS[69] and the other the

---

[68] Remember, we are concerned with where *drivers* are. A structural circuit per se is only a driver if there is reentry around that circuit.

[69] More precisely, "the" HPS wave is actually many parallel waves which spread down its various branches.

accessory pathway. Some ventricular cells are "under the influence" of the wave emerging from the accessory pathway, while others are under the influence of the wave(s) emerging from the HPS. Importantly, due to refractoriness, any given cell can be under the influence of only one wave.[70] We can think of the AVN and HPS as the *source*[71] of the passive waves they generate.

Where waves collide

Whether they've been generated by a single source (i.e. wave break) or two separate sources, waves can interact with each other. Initiation of orthodromic reciprocating tachycardia is a relatively straightforward example of what can happen when two waves interact: the wave front of the PAC

collides with the wave tail of the prior sinus beat (in the accessory pathway), causing unidirectional block and initiating reentry (Figure 60).

Waves can be generated in an ongoing fashion (as opposed to a single PAC). How will these interact?

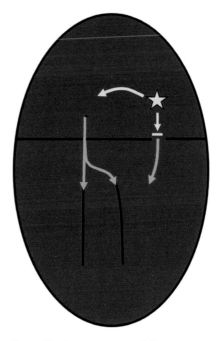

Figure 60 A premature atrial contraction (PAC) causes unidirectional block. A PAC delivered following a sinus wave (blue arrows). If pacing (star) is delivered closer to the accessory pathway than the atrioventricular node (AVN) activation (yellow arrows), it can block in the pathway and conduct through the AVN (if the conduction time from the pacing site to the node is sufficient to allow the node to recover from refractoriness).

---

[70] There is an uncommon and interesting exception: when there is a very large difference in conduction time via the fast and slow AV nodal pathways, a single sinus wave can travel via both the fast and slow pathways, producing two ventricular beats for a single atrial beat. To do so requires that the final common pathway (where the fast pathway and slow pathway waves meet in the distal AVN/proximal His) recover from refractoriness due to the fast pathway wave prior to the (very slow) slow pathway wave arriving.

[71] Here we are referring to *drivers* as the source of waves. Don't confuse "sources" in this context with current sources in the source-sink relationship. A wave source can be anything: the sinus node, a reentrant circuit, a pacing lead….

Two wave sources at the same rate

Waves emitted by two sources will propagate and collide somewhere between the two sources. If the sources produce waves at the same rate, those waves will travel the same distance each time before colliding, and hence the collision site will remain stable over time (Figure 61).

Two wave sources at different rates

If the two wave sources are producing waves at different rates, the faster source will send out waves progressively earlier relative to the slower source.[72] As a result, the wave from the faster source will travel farther than the wave from the slower source (it started its trip sooner), and the two waves will collide closer to the slower source. It is a truism that waves generated by two sources at different rates will collide *progressively closer to the slower source.* Another way to put this is that the region of cells under the influence of the fast source is progressively larger, while that of the slower source is progressively smaller (Figure 62).

Sources with variable rates

What if one of the sources is at a fixed rate but the other source (e.g. multi-wavelet reentry) produces waves at a variable rate, sometimes faster and sometimes slower than the fixed-rate circuit? If the variable source is faster, its waves will begin to collide *closer to the fixed-rate source.* But as its rate oscillates and becomes slower than the fixed-rate circuit, the wave collision site will start to ebb *closer to the variable-rate source.*[73] Depending upon whether the rate varies more frequently than the time required for collisions to reach either source, they can simply oscillate on and on in this way. There will remain two drivers of electrical activity in the tissue, with the regions under the control of one or the other repetitively growing and then shrinking.

If the frequency of oscillation is slower than the amount of time required for one circuit to reach the other, the faster circuit can reach the slower. If the slower source is reinitiated (by unidirectional block produced by a wave emanating from the fast source), the process can then repeat, with one driver alternately terminating and reinitiating the other.

---

[72] If a train leaves Chicago heading east once per hour and a train leaves Cleveland heading west every 50 minutes, the second train leaving Cleveland starts its trip 10 minutes sooner than the second train from Chicago. The third train leaves 20 minutes sooner, etc.

[73] As you might imagine, with multi-wavelet reentry not only is driver rate varying, but waves are coming from different distances/locations and directions.

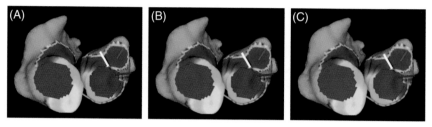

Figure 61 **Two wave sources at the same rate**. Counter-clockwise atrial flutter and left atrial pacing. Waves from both wave sources will repeatedly collide in the same location if pacing is at the same rate as tachycardia. A, B, and C are three sequential beats. *Source*: Modified with permission from [1].

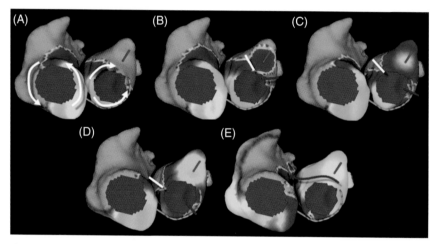

Figure 62 **Two wave sources at different rates**. (A) Counter-clockwise atrial flutter and (B–E) left atrial pacing. When paced rate is faster than tachycardia, waves from the two sources will collide progressively closer to the slower source (the atrial flutter circuit). Once the paced wave reaches the tachycardia circuit, there is only one source; everything is excited by the faster source (pacing). *Source*: Reproduced with permission from [1].

Source–source interaction: Who influences whom?

Wave sources can affect one another. Examples include overdrive suppression of slower pacemakers by faster ones, entrainment of reentry, and anti-tachycardia pacing. But sources cannot *directly* impact each other, they must **"communicate"** via the waves that they emit. That communication is in *one direction at a time*. Because waves can't travel through each other (due to refractoriness), source 1's wave can reach source 2 or vice versa, but not both. Before waves from the faster source have reached the slower source, there are two wave sources: some regions will be excited at the rate of the slower source and some at the rate of the faster. Once waves from the faster source reach the slower source, *all cells* are excited by the faster source – all cells are excited at the same rate.

To recap, drivers interact with one another via the waves they emit. Because waves cannot travel through each other, the interaction between drivers is one-way. Due to "starting their trip sooner each time," the waves from faster drivers will reach (and thereby can impact) slower drivers; not vice versa. When waves from the faster driver do reach the slower, the impact they have depends upon the mechanism of the slower driver (e.g. structural reentry, focal rotor). The faster driver can entrain or terminate the slower driver; in either case the faster driver is the *only* driver. The faster driver can de-anchor the slower driver, which, due to the dynamics of movement of variable distances according to location, is likely to result in the slower driver relocating to the faster region... where the tissue properties would result in the slower driver speeding up. Pretty much however you slice it, faster drivers dominate slower drivers.

PART III

Working with incomplete information

It seems reasonable at this point in the story to take a step back and ask what we do with all this information. In the face of competing hypotheses, (seemingly) contradictory data, and limited ability to *see* what is causing atrial fibrillation (AF) in an individual patient… what should we do with the person who's going to be on the electrophysiology lab table *tomorrow*? This is not an uncommon place to find oneself in the field of medicine: doctors virtually always have to make a concrete decision in the absence of complete information.

Much of the data we've reviewed is from animal models, where there is plenty of information available to determine specific mechanisms. The human data we've discussed is mostly from robust epicardial mapping performed in an operating room. Clinical electrophysiologists don't have access to this much data. The tools available at the time of writing this book have distinct limitations. It behooves us to understand what electrograms and mapping data actually tell us, so we can avoid jumping to erroneous conclusions from our maps.

Cardiac mapping

Cardiac mapping is a *sampling* problem. There is some objective information that we desire (in our case, the spread of electrical activation through the heart) and we would like to determine that information without acquiring *all* of the original *signal*.[1] If we want to

---

[1] There are different types of sampling, each with their own issues, but we can glean an appreciation for the relevant issues without getting too deep in the weeds.

Understanding Atrial Fibrillation, First Edition. Peter Spector.
© 2020 John Wiley & Sons Ltd. Published 2020 by John Wiley & Sons Ltd.

(A) (B) (C)

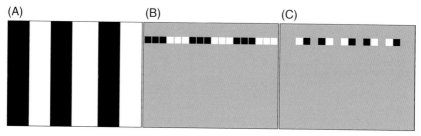

Figure 63 Sampling requirements: information vs. data. (A) If we would like to reconstruct a picture of vertical bars, (B) by sampling, (C) we need only sample at sites where colors change. Multiple samples from regions without change are redundant and not required to accurately reproduce the original image.

know how excitation spreads through the heart, can we measure the activation timing of some subset of cells to deduce the activation of the whole set *without* making an error?

Sampling and interpolation

This question (in a completely different guise) was addressed by Claude Shannon, the father of information theory. He was basically trying to determine *how little data* could be sent over phone lines *without loss of information*. The key to understanding his great insight is to focus on the distinction between **data** and **information**. Let me try to describe this using an example. Imagine a picture of white and black bars (Figure 63A). If we try to build a "map" of this picture by taking small, square samples (Figure 63B), we actually acquire *more* data than we need. In reality some of these data points (squares) are redundant; we really only need to

sample where there are *changes* in the picture color (Figure 63C). Shannon realized that if we record *all* the sites of change then everything *between* our samples (by definition) is unchanged. We can therefore reconstruct the original picture using only the samples we acquired. Of all the data that we could sample, the sites of change are the minimal set of samples we can acquire without loss of information (since we have all we need to accurately reconstruct the original "signal").[2]

You probably learned about this in the context of echocardiography, as the Nyquist sampling theorem. The theorem relates to the minimum frequency of sampling required to accurately determine the frequency of a signal. We typically employ the sampling theorem with time-varying signals, but it holds for spatially varying

---

[2] Summary: change equals information.

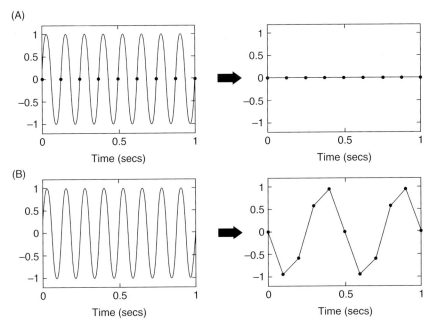

Figure 64 Sampling requirements: sample frequency vs. signal frequency. In order to accurately identify the frequency of a signal (sine wave), we must sample it at at least twice the frequency of the original signal. (A, left) If we sample at the same frequency, we collect data at the same amplitude with each data point (A, right) and wrongly conclude that there is no periodicity to the signal. If we sample at a rate greater than the signal but less than twice the signal frequency (B, left), we produce a time-varying signal, but not at the correct frequency (B, right). *Source*: Reproduced with permission from [83].

signals as well.[3] Forgetting the math, the gist of the matter is that in order to determine the frequency of a signal, we must make measurements of at least twice the frequency of that signal. This is easiest to appreciate with a sine wave (Figure 64). For a 2D image, this means that in order

not to lose information, one must make a measurement at least as often as there are changes in the underlying "signal."

What happens when we under-sample a map? The term for error introduced by under-sampling is **aliasing**. Aliasing refers to the erroneous introduction of "signal" that wasn't in the original image. In Figure 65, if we acquire data only at the sites of the red dots, we might

---

[3] It doesn't matter if we are looking at a sine wave relating amplitude to time or amplitude to distance – it's still a sine wave.

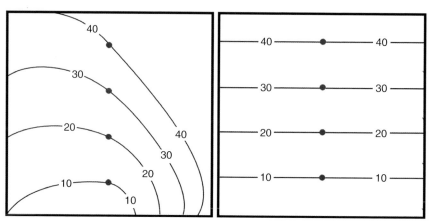

Figure 65 Aliasing in two-dimensional sampling. Aliasing refers to the erroneous introduction of "signal" not present in the original image. When we under-sample (red dots) asymmetrical, curved isochronal lines (left), interpolation produces an image with incorrect isochrones (right).

reasonably imagine that we have a planar wave propagating from the bottom of the tissue to the top (Figure 65 right), but in fact the underlying isochronal activation pattern is that seen in Figure 65 left. The erroneous isochronal lines are aliasing (inappropriately placing signal where there was none in the original).

In electrophysiology we aren't used to talking about Nyquist sampling or aliasing, but we are used to talking about number of map "points" and **interpolation**. When we make a 3D electro-anatomic map, we are basically creating an isochronal image (our map) from samples of an "original" (actual activation). The mapping system will often provide us with a map image that

has colors[4] *everywhere*, even though we only acquired data in a limited number of locations (Figure 66).

In order to fill in the "blank spots," the system performs a procedure called interpolation. Basically, it makes up colors to put *between* the data points. How does it decide what colors to use? Without any information, the system makes the assumption that the colors (activation timing) vary *uniformly* between data points. While this is a reasonable approach,[5] it is particularly misleading in cardiac

---

[4] Typically, activation time is color coded so our map isn't covered in numbers.
[5] With no additional information, what basis would we have for making any other assumption?

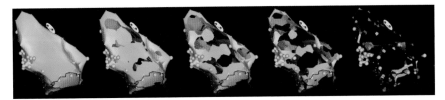

Figure 66 **Interpolation in three-dimensional electro-anatomic mapping**. Commercial mapping systems interpolate color between data points. Progressively reducing the interpolation distance makes the actual data distribution more obvious.
Source: Reproduced with permission from [11].

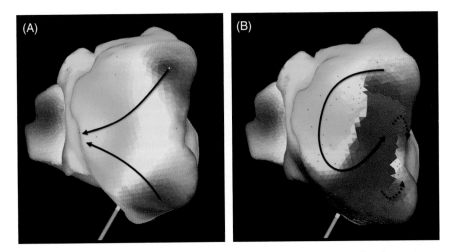

Figure 67 **Sample density and map accuracy**. (A) When we acquire too few data points (indicated by black dots), activation of the right atrial (RA) free wall appears to be from the annulus toward the posterior RA (arrows). (B) In reality, further data points indicate that there is counter-clockwise activation around a RA free wall scar (the scar is inferred by the activation pattern, not directly seen). We can also infer that there is a second vertical RA free wall scar closer to the annulus, revealed by activation around the top and bottom of the scar (dashed arrows). *Source*: Reproduced with permission from Visible Electrophysiology LLC.

mapping. When trying to understand an arrhythmia, it is generally true that the areas of interest are sites of *abrupt* changes in activation. So, in effect, interpolation is specifically misleading at the locations we are most interested in. The solution: *get more data points* (Figure 67).

In order to think through the issues that constrain this process, it is useful to introduce an analogy.

The image processing analogy for cardiac mapping

Imagine that the distribution of currents on the heart is plain to see; for example, because we are performing optical mapping where cell voltages are visible as colors.[6] *But* we can't look directly at the heart. Instead, we have to take a photograph of the heart and look at the picture to determine the distribution of colors.[7] The **sample density** is the number of pixels in our camera (which, in this analogy, is the analog of the number of electrogram recording sites). If we use a camera with two pixels we won't be able to discern much. However, if we use a 10 mega-pixel camera, we should have enough data samples to accurately reconstruct the original signal. There is a caveat: if our lens is out of focus, we *still* won't be able to tell what we're looking at. **Focus** in a photographic image is directly analogous to electrode **spatial resolution** in electro-anatomic mapping. Poor focus in an image causes blurring; colors from adjacent sites "bleed" into each other. In electro-anatomic mapping, currents from one location alter the potential field over adjacent locations. Thus, an electrode records an electrogram (the potential field) which is influenced by the cells *beneath* and *surrounding* the electrode. An electrode's spatial resolution can be thought of as the size of the area that contributes to the electrogram.

Sample density and sequential mapping

So, according to the Nyquist sampling theorem, we need to acquire a sufficient number of data points, close enough together, to accurately reconstruct the underlying activation pattern. The number that is "sufficient" depends upon the complexity of the activation pattern. When propagation is smooth (no changes in conduction velocity), then interpolation (which assumes no changes in conduction velocity) will be accurate. We require data points wherever there are changes in conduction velocity (rate or direction).[8] Thus the more complex

---

[6] A colleague of mine, Jason Bates (a lung mechanics maven, not an electrophysiologist), came up with this analogy.

[7] An optical map is actually a map of voltage not current, but it is the voltage gradients across the outer surfaces of cells that produce the currents that produce the potential fields we measure during mapping.

---

[8] Conduction velocity is a vector, i.e. it has amplitude and direction. Thus the required data (information) is any site at which amplitude and/or direction changes.

the rhythm, the more closely spaced our data points must be. It is often the case that the number of data points required is greater than the number of electrodes we can practically place in the heart. So then, how do we acquire a sufficient number of data points? The answer is we cheat. We perform *sequential* data acquisition. If the activation pattern is the same every beat, we can choose a reference electrode and acquire data sequentially across the chamber (measuring activation time relative to the reference signal). This turns out to be a particularly problematic issue for mapping of AF, but before we address that, we have one more piece of the mapping story to review.

Thus far we've been discussing mapping as if we directly measure the electric currents over each cell. In fact, that is not what we do.

Currents sources and potential fields

There is an important distinction between the electrical events that we are trying to deduce when we make maps and the thing we *measure* to construct maps. The former is *current* flowing at specific sites in the heart, while the latter is the *electric potential* generated by these currents. What's the difference? And who cares? The critical difference is that while the currents are spatially

discrete events,[9] the potential field that they generate spreads through space. The spreading of the potential field surrounding a current is directly analogous to the spread of the gravitational field surrounding a mass. While mass is at a specific location, it generates a gravitational field that spreads outward in all directions. The *magnitude* of this field diminishes with distance. This gives us a starting point for *working backward from the field measurement to the current distribution that generated it.*

This process of working backward (deriving the current distribution from measurements of the potential distribution) seems pretty straightforward. Surely with a formula and a calculator we should be able to determine *exactly* what the current distribution is… right? Sadly, no.

There *is* a formula that relates current to potential field. If we know

---

[9] Cardiac mapping seeks to identify how waves of electrical excitation propagate through the heart. These events (sequential excitation of myocytes) are local electrical events. By this I mean that while waves propagate through the atria, the events that comprise the waves are activation of cells which aren't moving at all. This is analogous to a sign in Times Square: we see words and images traverse across the sign, but this is really just a sequence of stationary lights going on and off in patterns. Similarly, for that matter, waves in the ocean are simply water molecules sequentially moving up and down; the waves move laterally, but the water only moves vertically (pretty much).

the size of the current, the distance between the current and the measurement location,[10] we can calculate the potential field *at that location* exactly. This is called the **forward problem**, forward because we are calculating the potential from knowledge of the current. The **inverse problem** is the opposite calculation, deriving the current from knowledge of the potential. The relationship between electric potential and the current that generates it is "non-unique." By this we mean that more than one distribution of current amplitude/location can generate the same potential.

Let me explain using mass and gravity rather than current and potential. Imagine that we cannot measure mass; instead, we have a tool for measuring the magnitude of the gravitational field (a scale). If our scale tells us that there is a "pull" of a given force (in a given direction), we can't say whether it is due to a bowling ball, 10 ft away, or a planet, 10 million miles away. In fact, the measurement could be due to an infinite number of combinations of masses and distances. Wait, says the clever student.[11] We can make *another* measurement from 20 ft in the direction of the pull. If the mass is a planet (farther in that direction), this second measurement will be larger[12] and from the same direction as the first measurement. Whereas, if the gravitational pull is due to a bowling ball only 10 ft from the first measurement site, then the second measurement will indicate a pull of the same magnitude as the first but in the opposite direction! This is very good. We *can* decrease the uncertainty of our deduction by making measurements at more locations. In fact, it would be pretty easy if there were simply one current source generating our field; in cardiac electrophysiology there is a very complex 3D distribution of current sources.

If you do the math, it turns out that you *can* calculate the exact distribution of currents that generated a given potential field – *if you make an infinite number of measurements.*[13] Measurements in this case refer to electrogram recording sites; so we need a lot of recording sites. With multi-site simultaneous mapping (e.g. epicardial electrode arrays), the number of recording sites equals the number of electrodes.[14] With sequential

---

[10] And an obscure measure of how easily the potential field is transmitted through space ("the permittivity of free space").

[11] …who is actually paying attention to this story.

[12] We are measuring a little closer to the planet.

[13] For those not mathematically inclined, that's a lot of measurements.

[14] Number of sites equals number of electrodes if we are making unipolar recordings; with bipolar recordings the number of measurements equals half the number of electrodes.

mapping, the number of measurements depends upon how many "points" we take; the number of measurements is not limited by the number of electrodes used.[15]

If we do not perform the inverse solution (if we simply look at the potential field), we are effectively looking at a blurred image of the current distribution. This is a subtly different issue from the issue of sampling and interpolation; increasing the number of samples doesn't solve this problem. Let me explain by analogy.

Who cares about spatial resolution?

Maps don't look blurry regardless of the resolution of your electrodes, so what am I carrying on about? We don't directly make maps with our electrodes; we record electrograms. We examine the electrogram to determine when a wave of activation has traveled beneath our electrode. We take *this* information ("local activation time") and place it at the location of our electrode on a 3D representation of the heart. The issue with spatial resolution (in this regard) is its impact on our ability to accurately determine the local activation time. If you think of an electrode as

"seeing" for some distance away from the cells immediately beneath it, the area that the electrode sees is its recording region. If there is organized propagation (often not the case in AF), it doesn't particularly matter if the electrode records from a region of 1 cm or 1 mm. Either way, there is a single discrete deflection on the electrogram which can provide an estimation of the local activation time.[16] The problem arises when the cells within the electrode's recording region are activated *dyssynchronously*. As electrical remodeling in AF progresses, activation grows ever more spatially complex [47, 49, 85]. There is a perturbation in the potential field every time any bundle of cells within the electrode recording region is activated; this means there is a deflection on the electrogram *for each* asynchronous group of cells activated. This can produce what are called "complex fractionated atrial electrograms" (CFAE; Figure 68) [86].

How do we decide which deflection represents local activation time? The reality is that they *all* reflect local activation time; the problem is that *local* is not local enough.

---

[15] Number of points equals number of electrodes × number of times we acquire local activation time with those electrodes.

[16] There is a lot that can be said about how to determine local activation time from an electrogram (whether unipolar or bipolar). We don't particularly need to delve into that story here. For those interested, see [84].

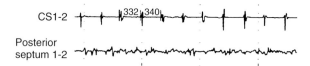

Figure 68 Complex fractionated atrial electrograms. Organized signal from the coronary sinus (CS1-2, top tracing) in which cycle length can easily be measured. Compare with the fractionated signal from the posterior septum (lower tracing) in which local activation time is ambiguous. *Source*: Reproduced with permission from [86].

Fractionation results from inadequate spatial resolution

CFAE are used by some clinicians to guide AF ablation [86–89]. But we and others have demonstrated that fractionation is a non-specific finding. *Any* cause of dissociation in the excitation of the cells in an electrode's recording region will produce fractionation [85, 90, 91]. Fractionation has been demonstrated to result from "zig-zag" propagation through infarct scar [92, 93], in areas of slow conduction due to fibrosis [90, 94], at the junction between focal rotors and the surrounding region of wave break [85], at sites of wave collisions, and during meandering of a rotor [91, 95]. There are multiple causes of dissociation that do *not* reflect AF drivers (e.g. wave collision). We demonstrated that fractionation results from mismatch between the size of an electrode's recording region (its spatial resolution) and the distance over which electrical activity is dissociated (tissue spatio-temporal frequency) [96].

If the electrode resolution is improved such that it "sees" an area of tissue small enough that all cells in that region are synchronously activated, there is no fractionation. Thus, because AF increases spatio-temporal frequency, spatial resolution must be increased to avoid fractionation (Figure 69).

Dominant frequency mapping

Some investigators have side-stepped the problem of ambiguous local activation time (fractionation) by examining electrograms in the *frequency domain* instead of the *time domain*.[17] The time domain refers to voltage versus time (a standard electrogram view). The frequency domain examines the frequency content of the deflections without regard for *when* in the signal that content

---

[17] Berenfeld has demonstrated that even when electrograms are discrete (i.e. there is a discernable local activation time), cycle length mapping can be a less accurate reflection of rotor frequency than DF mapping [97].

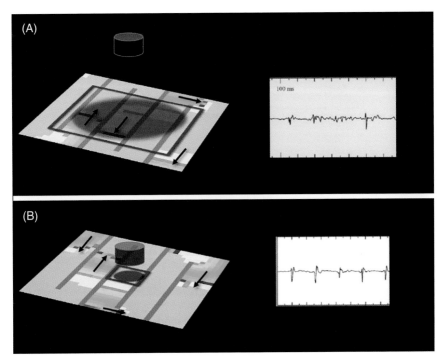

Figure 69 Spatial resolution and electrogram fractionation. Spatio-temporal variation was created as zig-zag activation through tissue with alternating linear ablation lesions (arrows, left). (A) When an electrode is high above the tissue, it "sees" multiple channels of propagation and hence generates a fractionated electrogram (right). (B) When the electrode is placed closer to the tissue surface, it "sees" a smaller region (one channel) and hence generates an organized electrogram (right). *Source*: Reproduced with permission from Visible Electrophysiology LLC.

arises (Figure 70). For more on dominant frequency (DF) analysis, see Appendix B. For the purposes of this discussion, what matters is that this doesn't entirely overcome the problem. Without delving into the details,[18] DF mapping does a pretty good job as long as the electrogram is

regular (periodic) and has consistent amplitude. The chaotic nature of fibrillation often means that activation isn't periodic. It also means that waves are traveling in varying *directions*. Direction matters, in the context of this discussion, because when mapping with bipolar electrodes, electrogram amplitude varies depending upon the difference

---

[18] See Appendix B.

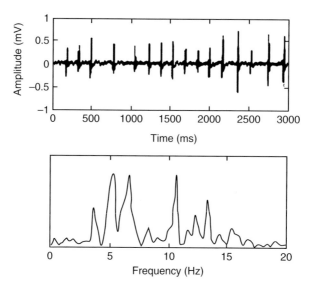

Figure 70 Dominant frequency analysis of electrograms. Dominant frequency analysis (bottom) captures the frequency content of electrograms (top). The power spectrum (frequency vs. power) quantifies the magnitude of the contribution of various frequencies during the period recorded. There is no information about when the frequency components occurred within the signal (e.g. the power spectrum would be identical if the electrogram were reversed in time). *Source*: Modified with permission from [83].

between the *direction of the wave* and the *axis between the electrodes* (of a bipolar pair; Figure 71).[19]

Spatial resolution and electrogram frequency

We examined the impact of electrode resolution on the accuracy of frequency maps during fibrillation. We tested the ability of electrogram frequency mapping to identify driver regions during multi-wavelet reentry. In a series of computational modeling experiments, we induced multi-wavelet reentry with burst pacing in 2D sheets of myocytes. Within these tissues, we created a short wave length patch, a region where cells had shorter action potential duration (APD). When we tracked the movement of circuits across the tissue, we found that circuit cores tended to congregate in these short APD patches. When we measured the frequency of cellular activation (number of action potentials per minute), it was highest in these patches (Figure 72). We also calculated the electric potential field surrounding the tissue, so we could calculate electrograms and perform mapping.

---

[19] See Section 3.1.9.2.

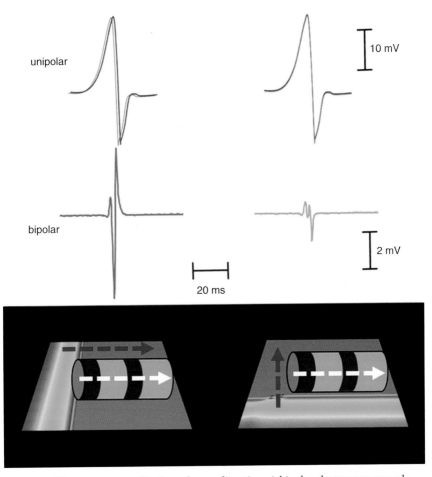

Figure 71 Electrogram amplitude and wave direction. A bipolar electrogram records the difference in the potentials recorded at both electrodes. If a wave is traveling in the same direction (red arrow) as the axis between the electrodes (white arrow), the unipolar electrograms (top left) are offset in time and the difference signal (middle left) has larger amplitude compared with a wave whose direction is perpendicular to the axis between the electrodes (right). In this case the unipolar electrograms are superimposed (right top) and hence tend to cancel each other out in the difference signal (right middle). Because the unipolar electrograms are not identical, the perpendicular electrogram is not completely flat. *Source*: Modified with permission from [1].

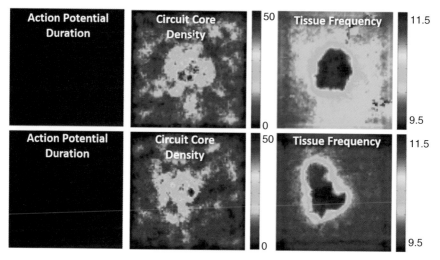

Figure 72 **Tissue wave length, circuit core density, and tissue activation frequency during multi-wavelet reentry.** In computational modeling of 2D sheets of cells, randomly shaped patches of cells with reduced action potential duration were included (red patches, left). Multi-wavelet reentry was induced and circuit core density was measured (middle). Cores were more often found in short wave length patches. When the activation frequency of each cell was recorded (right), the short wave length patches were easily identified as being excited at a faster rate. *Source*: Reproduced with permission from [98].

Electrogram frequency mapping

Using electrodes of varied spatial resolution, we made multiple frequency maps of the same episode of multi-wavelet reentry. We then calculated the correlation between the electrogram frequency maps and the actual cellular activation frequency distribution. The *tissue* activation frequency correlated with circuit core density, revealing the region driving multi-wavelet reentry. However, the accuracy with which the *electrogram* frequency map correctly identified the high-frequency tissue region (the region of high circuit density) varied tremendously with spatial resolution and the degree of electrogram fractionation (Figure 73).

Thus, while tissue frequency maps identify circuit cores, electrogram frequency may not. When spatial resolution was inadequate, dyssynchrony in the recording region created fractionation. When this occurred, electrogram frequency was *higher* than the frequency of activation of any individual cell (overcounting). If the spatial resolution is

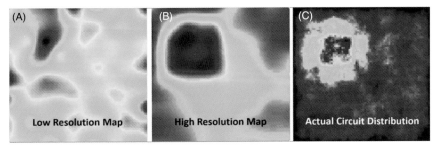

Figure 73 Frequency mapping as a function of electrode spatial resolution. Circuit core density (C) was measured during multi-wavelet reentry in a sheet of tissue with a square short wave length patch. Electrogram frequency maps were recorded using electrodes with low (A) and high (B) resolution. The location of the high circuit density region is much more clearly identified using high-resolution electrodes. *Source*: Reproduced with permission from [98].

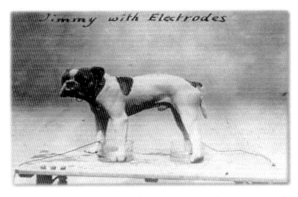

Figure 74 Early electrocardiogram (EKG). Via a string galvanometer, saline-filled dishes are used as electrodes to record an EKG from Jimmy.

increased such that all the cells in the electrode's recording region are activated synchronously, then there is only one deflection per cell activation, and tissue frequency equals electrogram frequency.

We therefore sought to create electrodes with sufficient spatial resolution to produce organized signals during AF.

What determines spatial resolution?

The first recording of cardiac electricity was the electrocardiogram (EKG; string galvanometer). The EKG measures the potential at the body surface (Figure 74).[20] While the EKG was a huge step toward understanding

───────────────

[20] In this case at the paws.

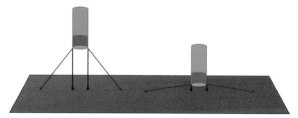

Figure 75 Spatial resolution and electrode height. Intracardiac electrodes have better spatial resolution (ability to distinguish signals directly beneath the electrode from those remote from the electrode). Electrogram amplitude diminishes as the distance between electrode and current source increases. Therefore, placing an electrode closer to the heart surface increases the distance discrepancies between "near" and "far" current sources. Thus closer cells contribute more to the electrogram than cells farther away.

cardiac electricity, it has very low spatial resolution; with a single lead you can "see" activation of the entire heart (P wave and QRS). Much later, intracardiac electrodes were used; these had the advantage that they helped distinguish the activation of the region underneath the electrode (near field) from activation of more distant regions of the heart (far field). How does this work? What is *near* versus *far* field?

The potential field diminishes with the square of the distance from the source current.[21] Thus an electrode registers its largest signal in response to activation of the cells that are closest.[22] By placing an electrode onto the surface of the heart, we alter the relative distances between cells and the electrode (Figure 75).

Electrode design and spatial resolution

We've said that spatial resolution is a measure of the size of the region that contributes to an electrogram. But there is no discrete edge to the "recording region." However, the impact of current on electrogram amplitude becomes negligible over varying distances as a function of several electrode properties. We quantified the impact of these characteristics

---

[21] This is a bit of an over-simplification, but it is adequate to accurately explain spatial resolution. For a more detailed discussion, see "What we measure when we measure electrograms" in [1].

[22] This makes the not entirely accurate assumption that the sizes of the sources (near and far) are equal. This is not true, for example, if "near" is thin atrial tissue and "far" is thick ventricular tissue.

on resolution [99, 100]. The first is the electrode's height above the tissue surface. The ability of intracardiac electrodes to localize current sources is due to the geometric relationship between the electrode location and the location of the electrical activity. When an electrode is high above the heart (e.g. with an EKG), it is roughly the same distance from all portions of the heart.[23] An electrode on the heart's surface is much closer to some cells than it is to other cells, therefore the "near" cells contribute much more to the electrogram than the "far" cells do.

Electrode size and shape have an impact on spatial resolution as well. Not surprisingly, a wide electrode, which covers a larger region of tissue, has a lower resolution than a narrow electrode (with a smaller "footprint"). It is not simply that the cells beneath the electrode are all equidistant from the electrode and hence contribute equally to the electrogram, but also that there is no way to distinguish *which* cells under the electrode generate the electrogram. Electrodes are conductors, hence there can be no voltage gradient on an electrode (current would immediately flow to dissipate the gradient). The consequence is that the potential recorded

by an electrode (the electrogram) is the mean of the potentials at each location on the surface of that electrode. Figure 76 helps to illustrate this point. We see a "finite element electrode" (FEM) above a narrow channel of propagation through a scar. The FEM electrode is equivalent to many small, closely spaced, square electrodes configured to create a large cylindrical electrode. However, the square "elements" are electrically insulated from one another; therefore, no current flows between them. First let's look at the bottom of the cylinder (touching the tissue). We can see that the part overlying the propagation pathway has a higher potential (red) than the part lying above the scar (green/blue). If this were not an FEM electrode, current would flow along the electrode from red to green, such that the electrogram amplitude would simply be equivalent to yellow. There would be no way to tell whether the pathway was beneath the near edge, the center, or the far edge of the electrode.

The thickness of the electrode (in Figure 76, the height of the cylinder) also affects resolution. Once again, the FEM electrode helps to illustrate why. The portions of the electrode that are farther from the tissue surface record a smaller potential (e.g. yellow) than the portions touching the tissue (red). If

---

[23] And therefore, all cells contribute (roughly) equally to the electrogram/EKG.

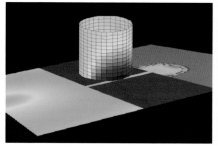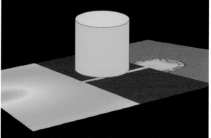

Figure 76 Finite element electrode. (Left) Here we see activation propagating from left to right across a narrow channel through scar tissue (gray). The finite element electrode (cylinder broken into many rectangular segments) is positioned so that one edge aligns with the channel, while the majority of the electrode sits above scar tissue. We can see that the portions of the electrode adjacent to the scar have the largest potential (red), and as elements are farther away the potential is diminished (yellow to blue/green). Potential diminishes with both height above the channel and lateral distance away from the channel. (Right) With an intact electrode (i.e. *not* a finite element electrode) there can be no gradient within the conductor and hence the potential reflects the average of the potentials that would be recorded by a finite element electrode. *Source:* Reproduced with permission from Visible Electrophysiology LLC.

this were not an FEM electrode, the currents would shift such that the electrogram would reflect the average potential over the entire electrode surface. It would be equivalent to a flatter electrode lifted off the tissue. Because the potential on the entire electrode is the same, there is zero spatial resolution over its surface (Figure 76) [99].[24]

Quantifying spatial resolution

In order to study the relationship between electrode design and spatial

resolution, we needed a way to quantify resolution. One measure is the "distance to half-maximal" amplitude (D½max), a measure of how far a current source is from the electrode when the potential it generates falls by half its maximum value. This is slightly less straightforward than it sounds. Unlike unipolar electrograms (Figure 77A), for bipolar electrograms, "max" is actually a negative value (Figure 77B). It is also worth pointing out that a bipolar electrode pair "sees" farther in the direction parallel to the axis between electrodes than perpendicular to it (Figure 71). It doesn't really matter; the idea is simply to have a consistent measure

---

[24] There is no way to distinguish between currents that arise from different locations *under* the electrode.

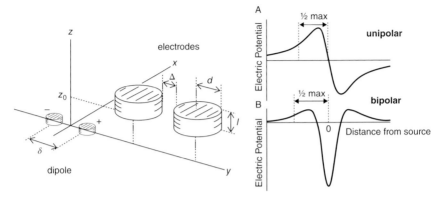

Figure 77 Quantifying spatial resolution: distance to half maximal amplitude.
A dipole source (small discs left) generates a potential field that is recorded by electrodes
(larger discs left) as the electrodes are moved progressively farther from the dipole source.
Electrograms (right) reveal amplitude as a function of distance (dipole to electrode(s)).
The spatial resolution is arbitrarily quantified as the distance at which electrogram
amplitude falls to half of its maximum deflection (for the bipolar signal the largest
deflection is downward). *Source*: Reproduced with permission from [1].

in order to compare between electrodes tested.

We were particularly interested in
the ability to distinguish near-field
from far-field electrical activity. We
therefore developed and tested a second measure of spatial resolution: the
distance between two current sources
at which they generate an electrogram
that is *most different* from a single
current source (Figure 78).

In a computational model, we
calculated the electrograms that were
measured as two sources were separated by 0–10 mm (Figure 78A). The
cross-correlation was then calculated
between the electrogram from superimposed sources (equivalent to a
single source) and those from sources

progressively farther apart.[25] The
correlation diminished as the sources
were separated, reaching a trough
and then increasing again as the two
sources became far enough apart to
generate two independent electrograms (Figure 78B). The spatial resolution was quantified as the distance
to minimum cross-correlation (C_{min}).

With a unipolar electrode of 1 mm
diameter, 1 mm thickness, and 1 mm
above the tissue surface, C_{min} = 4.5 mm
and D½ = 3.0 mm. When the diameter

---

[25] If two signals look the same (increased
cross-correlation) you can't distinguish them;
the distance between sources, where the signals are most different, is the distance at which
it is easiest to distinguish that there are two.

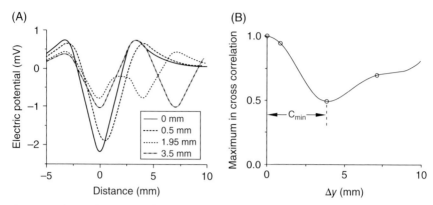

Figure 78 Quantifying spatial resolution: minimum correlation distance. Two dipole sources are used to generate a potential field. As the two dipole sources are moved progressively farther apart (from each other), the electrogram generated (A) is correlated with the electrogram from a single dipole (B). When the dipoles are superimposed, the signal correlates perfectly with a single dipole (and hence is indistinguishable). As the dipoles move farther apart, the correlation decreases to a minimum C_{min}. As the dipoles are moved farther apart, correlation begins to increase (as the second dipole gets too far to contribute significantly to the electrogram). The distance at which the electrogram correlation is lowest (C_{min}) is used as a measure of spatial resolution; it correlates with the location at which two different sources are most easily identified as being separate. *Source*: Reproduced with permission from [1].

and thickness were decreased to 10 µm (keeping height at 1 mm), $D\frac{1}{2}$ and C_{min} were reduced by an order of magnitude [99].

Recording configuration and spatial resolution

Electrodes can be configured to record bipolar or unipolar. Unipolar refers to a bipolar recording in which one of the two electrodes (the "indifferent" electrode) is far enough from the heart that it essentially records zero potential. Under these circumstances, a unipolar electrogram effectively displays only the potential of

the electrode in the heart (the "index" electrogram minus zero "equals" the index electrogram). Bipolar refers to a recording in which both electrodes are close enough to the tissue for each to be measuring a non-zero potential; the electrogram is the difference between the unipolar electrograms that would be recorded at each of the electrode sites. If the electrodes "see" the exact same thing, there is no difference and the electrogram is zero (a flat line). This has an impact on spatial resolution because as a source is moved farther away from a pair of electrodes, it looks ever more similar to both. Therefore, when you subtract one from the other, the difference decreases, i.e. far-field signals are small. As two electrodes are moved closer together (decreased interelectrode spacing), the far-field signals look more and more the same to each of them. Therefore, interelectrode spacing is inversely proportional to the spatial resolution of bipolar electrodes [99]. This capacity to diminish far-field signal enhances the effective spatial resolution of bipolar electrodes.

However, bipolar electrodes have a larger footprint than unipolar electrodes[26] and their amplitude is *direction dependent*. Direction dependence refers to the geometric relationship between the electrodes and a wave of excitation (the source). When a wave approaches along the direction of the axis between the electrodes, the distance between the source and each electrode is maximally different and the potential is largest. When a wave approaches perpendicular to the long axis between the electrodes, the source is at all times equidistant from both electrodes, hence the difference is zero; bipolar electrodes are blind to waves traveling in a perfectly perpendicular direction. Direction

independence is critical in AF mapping where waves travel in ever-changing directions. We therefore needed an electrode design that conferred high spatial resolution and direction independence.

Orthogonal close unipolar (direction independence and maximum spatial resolution)

We demonstrated that when a bipolar electrode pair is oriented "normal" to the plane of the tissue, it becomes direction independent and its spatial resolution is improved (compared with a contact bipolar; Figure 79) [100]. We call this orientation "orthogonal close unipolar" (OCU), because it is orthogonal to the tissue, only one electrode is in contact with the tissue (unipolar), and the indifferent electrode is very close. The impact of this geometric orientation is (i) reduced footprint, (ii) increased near-field–far-field discrimination), and (iii) direction independence (because the electrodes have the same geometric relationship to waves coming from any direction).[27] We assessed the ability to reduce far-field signal in swine heart by comparing orthogonal to contact bipolar electrodes (Figure 80). The ratio of far- to near-field signal was 0.15 ± 0.07 with contact bipolar recording versus 0.08 ± 0.09 with OCU

---

[26] The footprint is the area beneath the electrode. Unipolars have one footprint and bipolars have two.

[27] Except transmurally, through the tissue.

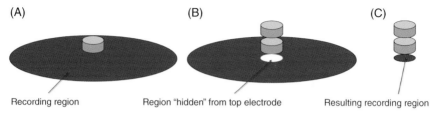

Figure 79 Orthogonal close unipolar recording region. (A) With a single electrode there is a large recording region extending laterally from the site beneath the electrode (gray circle) and diminishing with distance. (B) When a second electrode is placed directly above the first (orthogonal to the tissue surface), it largely "sees" the same recording region as the lower electrode, except it cannot "see" through the bottom electrode (white circle). (C) Therefore the difference signal (bipolar recording configuration between top and bottom electrode – "orthogonal close unipolar") "sees" only the area directly beneath the bottom electrode (small gray circle). *Source*: Reproduced with permission from Visible Electrophysiology LLC.

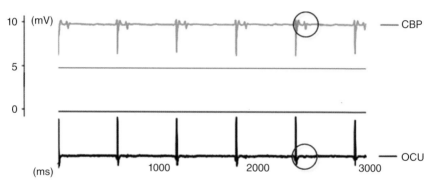

Figure 80 Improved far field cancellation using orthogonal close bipolar electrode configuration. Electrodes were placed epicardially over the atrium near the mitral annulus of a swine heart. Electrodes were configured as contact bipolar (top, CBP) and orthogonal close unipolar (bottom, OCU). The amplitude of the far-field ventricular signal is markedly reduced on the OCU recording (circled). *Source*: Reproduced with permission from [100].

recording (p<0.001), corresponding to a 53% reduction in far-field signal. The direction of wave propagation relative to electrode orientation had a significant impact on the amplitude of contact bipolar signals (7.6±3.7 mV parallel vs. 3.0±1.3 mV perpendicular; p = 0.001), while there was no change in the amplitude of the OCU signal (3.3±1.4 mV independent of wave direction) [100].

Sample density and atrial fibrillation

Now we return to the sampling problem. An electrode that has sufficiently *high spatial resolution* (to produce organized signals, with discrete, unambiguous, local activation time) *is necessary, but not sufficient* to map AF. We still need to solve the problem of acquiring a sufficient number of data points to unambiguously determine the mechanism(s) and location(s) of AF drivers.

The standard means by which electrophysiologists deal with sample density (i.e. number of map points) is to perform **sequential** mapping. The basic concept is that one builds up a map of local activation times *over many beats*. This can only be done *if the rhythm is the same every beat.* You simply leave one electrode in the same place throughout the map acquisition (the "reference" electrode) and compare the timing at all other sites to the timing at the reference site. This way one (or multiple) mapping electrode(s) can be moved around over many beats to piece together an activation map. Sequential mapping, by using the same electrode over and over, allows the number of points in the map to exceed the number of electrodes in the heart. Unfortunately, during AF atrial activation changes from beat to

beat and sequential mapping becomes meaningless.[28]

The inability to perform sequential mapping of AF has been doubly challenging. Not only is the number of points limited to the number of electrodes in the heart, but because AF is more spatially complex than organized rhythms, it actually requires *more* data points than an organized rhythm. Several approaches have been employed to deal with this.

Multi-site simultaneous mapping

In multi-site simultaneous mapping, sometimes called single-beat[29] mapping, one acquires all points at the same time. This has been done with catheters that have multiple, widely spaced electrodes. The idea is to get a (relatively) panoramic view of the atria. Some systems use a 64-electrode basket catheter, so electrodes are widely dispersed in a single chamber. Other systems use a large number of electrodes on the body surface and then perform the inverse solution (discussed earlier) to "project" electrograms

---

[28] It would be as if you tried to compile a picture of someone's face by taking pictures of small parts of their face and then gluing them together, except different people were photographed for each section. The collage wouldn't look like the original face or any *actual* face.

[29] Not because only one beat is mapped, but because *each* beat is mapped with all electrodes.

on the epicardial surface of the heart. The problem with these approaches is that the sample density is insufficient given the spatial complexity of fibrillation. Why don't these approaches suffer from inadequate spatial resolution? They do.

Sequential mapping of atrial fibrillation

There are some electrophysiologists who use alternatives to activation mapping. The idea is to identify AF drivers *without creating a complete activation map*. Several methods have been employed: CFAE mapping, DF mapping, and voltage mapping. In each case the presumption is that one need not create an activation map, or directly visualize drivers. We will examine each of these in turn. They share a common requirement: that the thing being mapped *is not changing* during the map (as a result, data can be acquired sequentially).

Complex fractionated atrial electrogram mapping

Fractionated electrograms have been identified in many rhythms (e.g. studies of atrial flutter, ventricular tachycardia, and in AF). As we've discussed, it has been repeatedly shown that anything that causes dyssynchronous activation within the recording region of an electrode produces fractionation. Having said this, Allessie's group sought to examine whether specific

electrogram morphologies could be correlated with the *type* of underlying activation. They performed high-density simultaneous multi-electrode[30] mapping (not easily achieved in the clinical setting) and then examined the morphology of individual electrograms (easily obtained) so as to correlate morphology with underlying activation pattern [101]. They meticulously created isochronal activation maps. Specific activation features were then identified: conduction block (defined as an activation difference of >30 ms between adjacent electrodes associated with a *change in direction* of activation distal to block), slow conduction (>30 ms time difference between adjacent electrodes, but with conduction in the same direction beyond the site of delay), pivot point ("the end of a line of functional block where the impulse makes a U-turn"), and collision (where electrodes were activated later than each of their neighbors; Figure 81) [101].

They detected single, "short" double (<10 ms interpotential difference), "long" double (10–50 ms interpotential difference), and fragmented signals ("multiple negative deflections"). They found that most long double electrograms were associated with a line of conduction block. At pivot points, where activation turned

---

[30] 244 electrodes, size not reported, interelectrode spacing 2.25 mm.

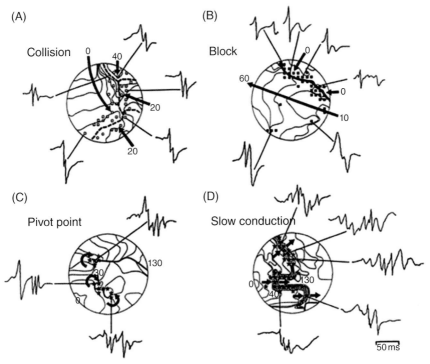

Figure 81 **Relationship between electrogram morphology and activation pattern**.
Epicardial electrograms were recorded from humans during atrial fibrillation. (A) Short
double electrograms were associated with wave collision. (B) Long double electrograms were
seen with conduction block (C and D) and fractionated signals were observed in association
with pivot points and slow conduction. *Source*: Reproduced with permission from [101].

around an area of block, electrograms were fragmented. Fragmentation was functional (during sinus rhythm there was no fractionation in these same locations; in fact, most complexes were single potentials even during fibrillation).[31] Approximately 50% of

fragmented potentials were associated with a pivot point. So, while fragmentation had a high negative predictive value (for slowed conduction or pivot points), it had poor positive predictive power [101].

Based in part upon the findings in that study, Nademanee hypothesized that by mapping CFAE (Figure 82) "it should then be possible to locate areas where the AF wavelets reenter. If such areas were to be selectively

---

[31] The fact that CFAE can come and go even when the electrode remains at the same location demonstrates that fractionation is a mismatch between tissue spatio-temporal variability and electrode spatial resolution.

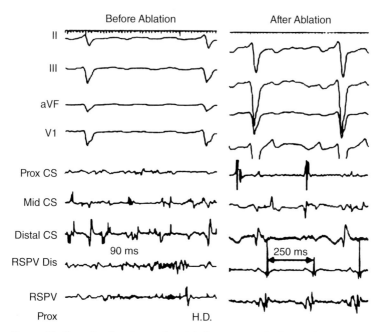

Figure 82 Complex fractionated atrial electrograms before and after ablation. aVF, Augmented vector right; DistalCS, distal CS electrogram; MidCS, mid CS electrogram; Prox CS, proximal CS electrogram; RSPVProx, proximal right superior pulmonary vein electrogram; V, voltage. *Source*: Reproduced with permission from [86].

eliminated by catheter ablation, wavelet reentry should stop, thereby preventing the perpetuation of AF" [86]. In 121 patients (57 paroxysmal and 64 chronic), CFAE ablation resulted in termination of AF in 95, and 91% were free of arrhythmias at 12 months (92 after 1 procedure and 18 after 2).

Reading through the subsequent literature that assessed the efficacy of CFAE-guided ablation is somewhat similar to watching a "Rocky Balboa" boxing match, with studies alternately showing excellent [102–107] or very poor results [108–111]. This is all too common in the AF ablation literature. It likely reflects, in part, the complexity of the rhythm itself, but, perhaps more importantly, may result from the inadequacy of using a descriptive definition of AF rather than a mechanistic one. These studies may very well be treating different populations that only appear to be comparable.

Dominant frequency mapping

Based upon the optical mapping studies performed by Jalife's group, several labs have investigated DF mapping clinically. An initial study by the Bordeaux group suggested that ablation at sites with high DF resulted in a decrease in AF cycle length (a measure of global AF rate), while non-DF sites had no impact [72]. There have been conflicting results regarding the spatial and temporal stability of DF sites [58, 60, 73, 112, 113] and the efficacy of DF-guided ablation [59, 114]. These discrepancies may reflect the role of electrode spatial resolution on the accuracy with which *electrogram* frequency mapping reflects actual *tissue* frequency [98, 100].[32]

Mapping fibrosis

We know there is a correlation between atrial fibrosis and AF [115]. We also know that fibrosis can play an arrhythmogenic role in multiple ways. Fibrosis can be dense, devoid of surviving muscle bundles. In this setting, it may form a macro-reentrant circuit (around the scar), but it doesn't play a role in AF [116, 117].[33] Patchy fibrosis contains small, tenuously connected electrical pathways which can promote fibrillation. In modeling studies, it has been demonstrated that there is a "sweet spot" between too much discontinuity (conduction failure) and too little discontinuity (normal conduction). In this intermediate zone there is rate-dependent appearance of fractionated signals and it is easier to

induce fibrillation [117, 118].[34] Several investigators have demonstrated that intercellular coupling plays an important role in fibrillation; it can cause wave break and rotation [119], stabilization/anchoring of drifting rotors [120, 121], and structural micro-reentry [44, 45]. It has been demonstrated that the extent of fibrosis (as identified by delayed-enhancement MRI) correlates with outcomes in AF ablation [122]. This stimulated interest in mapping the distribution of fibrosis as a guide to AF ablation.

There is debate about whether one can use electrograms to identify sites of fibrosis. There has been much enthusiasm for identifying fibrotic regions as those in which bipolar electrogram amplitude is below some threshold (typically 0.5 mV). In one study, low-voltage zones and fibrosis (identified on delayed-enhancement MRI) co-localized [123]. There have been other investigators who cast doubt on the ability of electrograms to identify drivers of AF via detection of fibrosis. It has been suggested that CFAE and low-voltage sites do not necessarily represent an *anatomic* abnormality (i.e. may not be fibrosis) because they are seen during AF but

---

[32] See Section 3.1.7.2.

[33] Reentry around a large scar can be too slow to (i) cause fibrillatory conduction or (ii) drive fibrillation if "unprotected" (see Section 2.6.2).

[34] In the setting of compromised electrical connections, there are multiple sites of tenuous source-sink balance. Under these conditions conduction can be rate dependent, setting up conditions for unidirectional block and reentry [117].

not sinus rhythm [124].[35] One group used a circular mapping catheter to identify rotational activity, and then correlated rotation with CFAE and low-voltage electrograms. Most CFAEs did not co-localize with rotors, although most rotor sites had CFAE (85%) or low voltage (23%) [125]. A similar approach to assessing the physiological role of low-voltage zones found no correlation between rotors identified by focal impulse and rotor mapping (FIRM) and low-voltage zones [126].

Multiple investigators simply tested the impact that low-voltage electrogram-guided ablation has on outcomes of AF ablation. Several studies have demonstrated improved outcomes when low-voltage zones were targeted in addition to pulmonary vein isolation [127–132]. Ablation was either directed at decreasing fractionation or encircling/isolation of fibrotic regions. Others have not found incremental benefit to the ablation of low-voltage zones [133].

Mapping rotors

In the last several years there have been attempts at directly mapping the rotors (or focal firing) that drive AF. Using a basket catheter and proprietary software, FIRM attempts to identify rotational (or centripetal) activation patterns [134]. Despite using a standard, low-resolution basket catheter (electrode size not reported), they attempt to distinguish local activation time despite fractionated electrograms based upon certain physiological assumptions, derived from prior monophasic action potential (MAP) studies. While initial results looked promising [134, 135], subsequent studies demonstrated poor results [136–138].

Mapping atrial fibrillation reconsidered

There seems to be nothing but obstacles that prevent adequate map guidance for AF ablation. Simultaneous multi-site activation mapping requires too many electrodes,[36] CFAE is non-specific, DF mapping is subject to errors introduced by applying Fourier analysis to sharp and varied signals, and scar mapping is non-specific, revealing anatomy without physiology.

Mapping AF has two specific hurdles: (i) poor spatial resolution results in fractionated electrograms (and hence ambiguous local activation time); and (ii) changing activation

---

[35] Although, as we've seen, this may be because tenuous electrical connections conduct during slow rhythms, but block at rapid rates.

[36] I.e. FIRM and CardioInsight (body surface mapping) employ too few electrodes, of inadequate resolution.

precludes sequential mapping (high resolution or not, we are never going to be able to get enough electrodes in the heart for simultaneous mapping). One question we could ask is whether we *require* a complete activation map to identify driver type and location. The premise of AF activation mapping is that if we see *all* activation, we can directly *see* drivers. For one thing, computational modeling suggests that this is not necessarily true; e.g. with multi-wavelet reentry, driver regions are not obvious even upon visual inspection. The physiology we discussed in the first part of this book indicates that driver distribution is not random: drivers are where they are *because of* regional heterogeneities in the tissue. This suggests the possibility that **if we could map tissue properties**, rather than activation, we could *deduce* where drivers are located.[37]

Why would tissue property mapping be any better than activation mapping? The big challenge with *activation* mapping of AF is that activation keeps changing, which means we can't perform *sequential* mapping. Tissue properties are different: they aren't changing. Sure, over time they change due to remodeling, but during the time frame of a map they aren't

changing. If tissue properties aren't changing, we can map *them* sequentially. This solves the sample density problem: *sequential mapping untethers sample density from the constraint of electrode number.*

What tissue property would we map? The property that determines where cores are distributed. Before we delve into details, let me introduce an analogy. This would be like trying to map the distribution of water on some irregular surface... *if you were blind to water.* You might argue that you don't need to see water to know where it will be. If you understand the dynamics of flowing water and how it interacts with the architecture of surfaces, you know that water flows downhill and collects in low spots (local minima).[38] So, we can "map" water simply by making a topology map; for this we don't need a water detector, we just need an altimeter. And we can create this map *sequentially* (how high is this spot, how high is *this* spot, etc.).

---

[37] After all, it is the tissue properties that determine where the drivers are in the first place.

[38] "Minima" meaning that water won't necessarily all flow to the very lowest point on a hill. If the hill is varied in slope with multiple peaks and valleys, water will pool wherever there is a local valley (this is why there can be pools up in the mountains). Once water hits one of these, it would have to go *up* in order to move on to an even lower place (this is called a "basin of attraction").

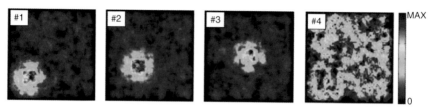

Figure 83 Circuit core density and short wave length patches. In a computational model, circuit core density was measured during multi-wavelet reentry. Cores co-localized with patch location; as the patch was moved from the lower left (1) to the middle (3) and in between (2), circuit core density increased at these locations. When there was no short wave length patch (4), circuits were homogeneously distributed. *Source*: Modified with permission from [82].

What, in cardiac tissue properties, is analogous to altitude in landscape properties? Multiple studies have demonstrated that in heterogeneous tissue, *drivers tend to be found in regions with relatively short APD/refractory period* [3, 39, 76, 139, 140].

We tested the hypothesis that drivers cluster in regions of short APD. Figure 83 shows tissue with a short APD patch: the plot indicates patch location and circuit core density distribution. The cores cluster where the patch is.

But how do we map APD? Catheter mapping is performed with extracellular electrodes, and electrograms reveal local activation time (the start of the action potential), but they do not reveal repolarization time (the end of the action potential). Thus, we can't directly see APD (the

time between activation and repolarization).[39] Here is where the chaotic nature of AF is actually an asset. In sinus rhythm, there is no relationship between APD and how often a cell is excited. In AF, there are

---

[39] There is an exception to this limitation. Michael Franz developed a particularly clever catheter design, the MAP catheter. This places a little force on the tissue beneath the tip electrode, which causes depolarization, inactivating sodium channels and rendering these cells unexcitable. The result is a voltage gradient between the cells beneath the electrode (fixed at a depolarized potential, e.g. -40 mV) and the cells surrounding the electrode. The surrounding cells rest at a lower voltage and rise to a more depolarized voltage when activated. As a result, there is a changing gradient that causes current flow (which the MAP catheter measures). The critical feature is that the time course of the gradient/current/electrogram *is determined by the APD* of the cells surrounding the MAP electrode. Thus, the MAP indicates the average of the APDs surrounding the MAP site.

chaotic waves propagating from every direction; *on average*, the limiting factor on how often a cell is excited by one of these waves is its refractory period. Areas with short APDs *can be* excited more often than areas with long APDs. If we can identify each time a cell is excited (which we can see with high-resolution electrograms), the **cycle length, during atrial fibrillation, is proportional to the local refractory period/APD**. While the absolute value of local cycle length may not equal the APD,[40] **the gradients in cycle length should still reflect the gradients in APD**. We don't care about the number (APD), we care about the *location* where that number is shortest.

Refractory period and cycle length during fibrillation

As we discussed in Section 3.1.7.2, we did a series of modeling studies to address this question. We created sheets of tissue with regional variations of APD (and hence refractory period). We induced multi-wavelet reentry in these tissues (with burst pacing) and measured circuit core

distribution. Circuit core[41] distribution correlated with regional gradients of APD (Figure 83) [82, 98]. We next measured the activation frequency of *each cell*. There was a distinct spatial correlation between the local APD and local *cell* cycle lengths (Figure 72) [98]. Thus, **circuit core distribution correlated with APD and with local tissue activation frequency**.

This is encouraging, but we need to be able to identify drivers *with electrodes* if we are going to guide clinical ablation. We therefore tested the hypothesis that electrogram frequency correlates with tissue frequency provided electrodes have sufficiently high spatial resolution to preclude fractionation. The logic is that a fractionated electrogram has a deflection every time *any cell in its recording region* is excited; if cells are excited dyssynchronously, electrogram frequency is *higher*

---

[40] If cells aren't excited as soon as they can be (i.e. if there is an excitable gap), then cycle length will be longer than APD.

[41] During multi-wavelet reentry, circuits can be spatially complex (not like the discrete core of a rotor). As a result, using phase singularities to identify cores misses some. We developed a different approach to core detection: we identified wave fronts, and thereby found free wave ends, which were tracked through space. When the wave end path crossed itself, the closed loop circumscribed was designated a circuit core. When we compared the wave end tracking with the phase singularity method (meticulous frame-by-frame visual inspection as control), wave end mapping had a higher sensitivity and specificity for circuit cores in multi-wavelet reentry [82].

than the frequency of any individual cell. In contrast, when a high-resolution electrode generates an unfractionated signal, it means that all the cells contributing to the electrogram are activated synchronously; hence the frequency of each cell is the same as the frequency of the group of cells and therefore of the electrogram. We measured the **correlation between electrogram frequency, tissue frequency, and circuit core density**. Correlation **improved as spatial resolution improved** (Figure 73) [98].

How is this any different from mapping DF? In principle it is no different; both seek to identify faster areas. DF mapping employs Fourier analysis to determine local activation rate. Unfortunately, Fourier analysis is not optimized for identifying the frequency of electrograms, particularly during AF. First, it is designed for sine waves, so the sharp morphology of electrograms requires processing in order to be "rounded" sufficiently to be amenable to Fourier analysis. Second, the accuracy of Fourier analysis

is diminished by variations in signal amplitude and frequency. Thus, the difference between prior studies of DF and our study is the *input*. By using high-resolution electrograms we improve our ability to detect cell activation rate, uncontaminated by asynchronous activation of neighboring cells (Figure 84).

DF mapping wasn't conceived to identify regional distributions of APD, it simply looks for the fast places. Is it sufficient just to look for fast places, regardless of whether those places have shorter APDs? For that matter, why do circuit cores localize in short APD patches? As we discussed in Section 2.7, the *extent* of meander is influenced by wave length. When wave length is long (relative to core size), the wave tip is more likely to interact with its own tail and meander. We also saw that in a random walk over landscape with a regional variation of step size, "walkers" will tend to cluster in short step-size zones. So, to the extent that meander distance is related to APD,

(A) (B)

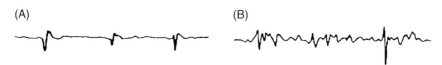

Figure 84 Local activation time and signal fractionation. (A) When electrograms have a discrete local activation time, Fourier analysis is not required, and one can directly measure cycle length. (B) With fractionated signals local activation time is ambiguous and Fourier analysis is required to identify frequency.

absent other influences, cores will tend to be concentrated in short APD regions. And, even if we ignore the meander piece of the story, we've seen that driver interactions are *unidirectional*. Faster drivers will interrupt slower drivers and hence the faster drivers… drive. Thus, (i) APD (via meander distance) and (ii) the impact of relative rate on driver predominance *both* suggest that faster regions are where we will find drivers in AF.

So, we propose that if we use high-resolution electrodes, we will minimize fractionation and, as a result, *electrogram* frequency will reflect local *cellular* activation frequency (without over-counting). With sharp electrograms, we don't *require* signal processing and Fourier analysis, we can directly measure the cycle length (frequency = 1/CL). Thus, high-resolution electrodes allow us to perform time domain[42] cycle length measurement. The chaotic nature of waves in AF means that cycle length correlates with refractory period (which correlates with circuit core density). And, regardless of the relationship between refractory period, cycle length, and cores, simply measuring *relative rates* should allow us to identify drivers.

Improving the sensitivity of tissue property mapping

We know that the physiology, and hence the distribution, of functional circuits is influenced by wave length, not simply APD. Because wave length is equal to the product of APD and conduction velocity, we considered the possibility that cycle length mapping might be less sensitive to gradients in wave length that are *due to gradients in conduction velocity*.[43] To test this, we modeled tissues in which APD was homogeneous, but there was a patch with higher intercellular resistance.[44] Figure 85 demonstrates maps based upon *tissue* conduction velocity, cycle length, and wave length. When there is a gradient in conduction velocity alone, cycle length mapping was much less sensitive than conduction velocity mapping (Figure 85). In contrast, when the gradient is in APD alone, cycle length mapping outperforms conduction velocity mapping. When we combine the two measurements to generate a wave length map, we detect gradients in either cycle length or conduction velocity.

---

[42] AKA normal electrograms.

[43] Rather than gradients of APD.

[44] Regional variation in conduction velocity alone, with homogeneous APD, is not particularly physiologically realistic, but gradients of conduction velocity *larger than* the gradient in APD might be.

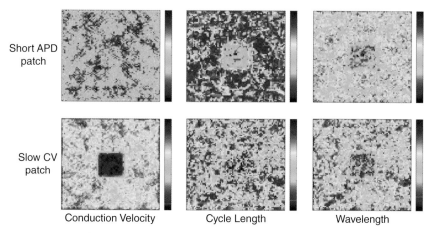

Figure 85 **Wave length mapping of fibrillation: tissue**. Fibrillation was induced (via burst pacing) in simulated tissues. There was a central patch with reduced wave length (relative to the surrounding tissue). Wave length was reduced by either decreasing action potential duration (APD, top) or increasing intercellular resistance, which decreased conduction velocity (CV, bottom). Maps were created of conduction velocity (left), cycle length (middle), and wave length (right) based upon cellular activation. Conduction velocity was more sensitive when gradients were due to intercellular resistance; cycle length mapping was more sensitive when gradients were due to variation in APD. Wave length detected the short wave length patch regardless of the etiology. *Source*: Reproduced with permission from Visible Electrophysiology LLC.

Wave length mapping with electrodes

We next examined whether we could use electrodes to identify wave length. We already know that with high-resolution electrodes (no fractionation), electrogram cycle length correlates with tissue cycle length. With the use of a 2D grid of high-resolution electrodes, we can estimate conduction velocity as well: the distance between electrodes divided by the time interval between their activations. This is only an estimate, because it *assumes* that conduction was directly between the electrodes (and velocity is constant). We can reduce error by placing electrodes very close together. Nonetheless, we are unlikely to align our electrodes with propagation at all times. There is no reason that the misalignment should vary from location to location and hence the error should be roughly the same everywhere. This suggests the possibility that *gradients* in conduction velocity will be accurately detected, even if the absolute values of the measured velocities are inaccurate. Figure 86 shows that we can map conduction velocity (and wave

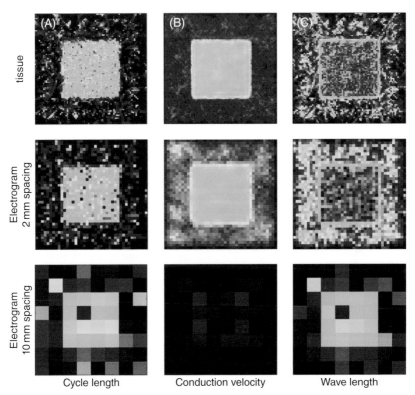

tissue

Electrogram 2 mm spacing

Electrogram 10 mm spacing

Cycle length   Conduction velocity   Wave length

Figure 86 **Wave length mapping of fibrillation: electrogram**. (A) Cycle length, (B) conduction velocity, and (C) wave length were mapped during multi-wavelet reentry. Maps were created, either directly, using tissue activation (top), or with electrodes (bottom). Map accuracy can be seen to vary with interelectrode spacing: 2 mm interelectrode spacing (middle), 10 mm interelectrode spacing (bottom). Note that conduction velocity accuracy diminishes as electrodes are moved farther apart. *Source*: Reproduced with permission from Visible Electrophysiology LLC.

length) with electrodes, and that, not surprisingly, accuracy is diminished as interelectrode distance is increased.[45]

---

[45] Note that cycle length measurement accuracy is independent of interelectrode spacing; each measurement is independent of other measurements.

But what kind of driver is it? distinguishing high circuit core density (in multi-wavelet reentry) from focal rotors

It is certainly critical to identify the location of drivers in order to ablate AF, but we also need to know which *type* of driver we are trying to ablate. The strategy for ablating moving circuits differs from that for ablating stationary circuits. The distribution of linear ablation for the treatment of moving circuits is guided by the probabilistic nature of meandering into boundaries. Stationary circuits require transection as well, but ablation must be delivered directly to the circuit (the circuits won't deliver themselves to the ablation). Identifying the fastest locations during fibrillation is sufficient to delineate these regions as drivers.[46] How do we tell which kind of driver?

We hypothesized that the regularity of activation distinguishes the two: rotors are periodic, while multi-wavelet reentry should have a much more variable rate. We created a series of tissues in which APD and conduction velocity were varied such that in some of the tissues burst pacing elicited focal rotors, while in others it produced multi-wavelet reentry. We then examined the activation time of each cell, and calculated the cycle length, conduction velocity, and *variability* of each of these (Figure 87). In Figure 87 there is a focal rotor in the top left corner of the tissue, with multi-wavelet reentry in the remainder of the tissue. Cycle length and conduction velocity mapping don't

clearly distinguish the focal rotor from multi-wavelet reentry, but analysis of variability clearly demonstrates a focal rotor in the top left corner of the tissue. In computational modeling of 2D tissue sheets, we examined 143 episodes of fibrillation. Focal and meandering rotors were identified in 113 tissues, and rotors were correctly identified via cycle length coefficient of variance, with a sensitivity of 0.86. There were no false positives, and false negatives primarily occurred in tissues with multiple meandering rotors.

What should we do with the patient who comes to the lab *tomorrow*? putting it all together (without "it all")

As is often the case, physicians find themselves in the position of treating patients with AF without adequate knowledge of what exactly is driving their patient's rhythm and where it is driven from. We are in a relatively fortuitous position given what we *don't* know. Despite the shortcomings, we actually have reasonably effective treatments for AF. While anti-arrhythmic medications work poorly, ablation is fairly effective [141]. We can cure some patients with AF, but ablation for fibrillation is far less successful than for most other

---

[46] Either a zone of high circuit core density in multi-wavelet reentry or the location of a rotor and the surrounding region in 1 : 1 continuity with the rotor.

Cycle length   Conduction velocity

Voltage

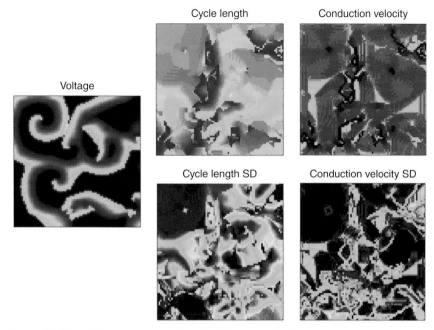

Cycle length SD   Conduction velocity SD

Figure 87 Variability mapping to identify driver type. Multiple maps of a tissue in which a focal rotor (top left corner of tissue) drives fibrillatory conduction in the surrounding tissue. (Left) Snapshot of voltage in a single time step. Focal rotor site is difficult to detect with cycle length (middle top) and conduction velocity (right top) maps, but is more apparent with cycle length variability (middle bottom) and conduction velocity variability (right bottom) maps. SD, standard deviation.

rhythms, with higher re-do rates and lower overall success.[47] It is only because anti-arrhythmics work so

poorly that ablation is the best treatment we have. The result is that we've had 20 years of experience placing catheters into the hearts of patients with AF. This has been a fantastic opportunity to learn.

First, do no harm: Ablation for AF has been driven all too often by fad; strategies tend to wax and wane in popularity. As a field we have not proven to be very analytic about our methods. Thus, perhaps step one in how to approach AF ablation in the

[47] There is a difference in the significance of reduced single-procedure success rate and that of overall success rates (independent of how many tries). Re-do procedures often mean that we have failed to achieve our strategic target, e.g. pulmonary vein isolation (PVI), in which case repeat procedures are aimed at simply succeeding at the initial plan. In contrast, limitations in the overall success rate indicate largely that the strategy itself was inadequate to cure AF.

setting of inadequate knowledge is to be a skeptic. When new techniques and strategies come out, consider whether or not they make sense, and whether the data support the claims.

Pulmonary vein isolation: Without question, the most consequential development in the field of AF ablation was the recognition by the Bordeaux group that AF is often triggered by rapid firing from the pulmonary veins. This ultimately led to the strategy of quarantining the pulmonary venous musculature from the atria. There is quite vast experience with this approach by now. The data suggest that pulmonary veins often trigger AF and that PVI is effective in about 75% of patients (with paroxysmal AF).

It is somewhat dangerous to draw *mechanistic* conclusions from the response to ablation. For example, PVI has many potential anti-fibrillatory effects. Quarantining the pulmonary venous musculature is certainly one. This may mean that elimination of pulmonary vein triggers is the crucial effect of PVI. But pulmonary veins often have multiple discrete atrial connections. This raises the possibility that the elimination of multiple micro-reentrant circuits contributes to PVI's anti-fibrillatory effect. It has also been demonstrated that there are numerous

autonomic inputs to the atria (the ganglionated plexi) located around the pulmonary venous ostia. We and others have demonstrated that during PVI and encircling, one can inadvertently destroy these plexi [142]. Since it has been well established that parasympathetic stimulation of the atria is pro-fibrillatory, it is quite possible that destruction of ganglionated plexi is (at least partially) responsible for the anti-fibrillatory impact of PVI.

What is clear, however, is that PVI often cures AF. Given that it is a fairly low-risk procedure, it is not a prerequisite that we know *why* PVI works.[48] Unfortunately, it is also quite apparent that PVI alone is not sufficient in all patients. It seems that *something* else is required, particularly in patients with more advanced AF.[49] A logical narrative that *could* apply is that early in the course of AF there is little structural or electrical remodeling and *initiation* of fibrillation is the problem; thus PVI is

---

[48] This is not to say that it wouldn't be desirable to know.

[49] Some have interpreted ablation studies that indicated no improvement, when additional ablation measures are added to PVI, as meaning that no additional ablation is required. That simply means that the particular additional lesions used in the study were inadequate. It seems clear that we do not have satisfactory ablation results in chronic AF, we "simply" need to determine *how* to identify what/where AF drives are, in a patient-specific manner.

pretty effective. Under these circumstances, "trigger elimination" is logical. One might even feel that by preventing AF, this approach precludes remodeling (AF "begetting" AF). It's important to recognize, however, that not only AF begets AF. Something else must beget it as well, or there would never be any AF in the first place.[50]

What about when pulmonary vein isolation isn't enough?

Success rates for ablation of persistent AF are lower than for paroxysmal AF. There are likely several explanations for this. First, not *all* triggers arise in the pulmonary veins. Unfortunately, it is quite difficult to find triggers. In fact, the best thing about PVI is that it obviates the need to find specific trigger sites; you simply quarantine all pulmonary venous tissue. Some researchers have proposed that AF triggers can arise in the superior vena cava (SVC), which suggests the possibility of leveraging the quarantine strategy here as well. There is a risk of causing damage to the phrenic nerve, so SVC isolation should be undertaken only with confirmation that SVC triggers are present.

Inadequate trigger elimination is not the only reason that PVI is sometimes insufficient. Due to structural and electrophysiological remodeling,

the atria's capacity to support fibrillation increases over time. Why is AF more stable with advanced disease? Is this due to a decreased refractory period and slowed conduction velocity, reducing wave length and increasing the number of circuits that the tissue can accommodate? Or is it because endomysial fibrosis creates micro-reentrant circuits that can drive AF? It is likely each of these contributes to various extents in most patients.

It is important to determine the *mechanism(s)* responsible for the perpetuation of persistent AF, because this will determine the appropriate ablation strategy. Various approaches have been advocated for how to alter atrial substrate. These include use of map identification of drivers (FIRM, CardioInsight, CFAE, DF) followed by *focal* ablation. Ignoring the veracity of mapping for a moment, what is the effect of focal ablation on a focal *reentrant* driver?

Impact of focal ablation on various driver types

Focal drivers can be non-reentrant (i.e. triggered or automatic), in which case destruction of the culpable cells is sufficient to eliminate firing. Drivers are often reentrant, either structural (micro-reentry) or functional (stable rotors). Micro-reentry results from a small structural circuit, which likely must be partially protected from the

---

[50] Perhaps it really *is* "turtles all the way down."

surrounding atrial tissue.[51] These circuits are small, so relatively focal ablation can be effective. In this setting, ablation that is not connected to an outer boundary may create a new structural circuit, but, because the resultant circuit would not be protected, it may not be a source for driving AF. Structural reentrant circuits need be protected only during fibrillation; it is the fibrillatory conduction from which protection is required. Thus, one *can* produce the substrate for atrial tachycardia with focal ablation (ablation not connected to a boundary). *Even with* partial protection, the ability of a structural circuit to drive *fibrillation* depends upon its size (path length), because slow reentry will be dominated by other, faster drivers.

Ablation of focal rotors

Rotors are functional reentrant circuits. Like all circuits, there are (and must be) two *separate* excitable paths connected at their ends. This is a somewhat convoluted way to describe the circular path of a stationary rotor, but it introduces a concept that is relevant to the ablation of rotors. Ablation at the center

of a rotor simply alters the way in which the circuit is structured, replacing the functional core with a structural core (the ablation lesion). Does this mean that focal ablation cannot terminate reentry driven by a rotor? No, there are several means by which focal ablation can terminate reentry at the ablation site. Focal ablation (i) can cause de-anchoring of rotors which can subsequently meander and terminate by colliding with a boundary; (ii) can result in a circuit too slow to participate in driving fibrillation; or (iii) if it creates a longer path length but an *even* longer wave length, the resulting circuit cannot support reentry (head meets tail) [35]. It is important to make the distinction between terminating an *episode* of tachycardia and *eliminating the capacity for reentry*. Obviously, our goal with ablation is to alter the atria's capacity to support fibrillation, not simply to terminate an episode. Otherwise DC cardioversion would be the cure for AF.

Putting it all together: Atrial fibrillation in three questions

What causes atrial fibrillation?

Anything that generates waves at a rate faster than can be conducted 1 : 1

---

[51] Based upon both biological findings in human ex vivo optical mapping and the principles of wave–wave interactions (see Sections 2.5 and 2.6.2).

to the entire atria causes AF.[52] The atria (and excitable media in general) are capable of supporting a wide array of different propagation patterns. These include stationary and moving circuits, each of which is a *reentrant rhythm*. The location(s) and rate(s) of these drivers are determined by complex interactions between cell physiology, tissue physiology, and tissue architecture, and dynamic interactions between drivers, mitigated by the waves they emit.[53]

How do we find the drivers of atrial fibrillation?

Using electrodes on trans-venous catheters, it is challenging to create activation maps that identify driver type and location. Limiting factors include (i) the spatial resolution of electrodes – inadequate resolution causes fractionated electrograms with ambiguous local activation time; and (ii) the need for high sample density and multi-site simultaneous panoramic recording, which mandates

more electrodes than can practically be delivered to the heart. One way to overcome these hurdles is to map local tissue activation properties (cycle length, conduction velocity, and their variability) using electrodes with high spatial resolution and direction independence. The latter can be achieved with the use of very small, thin, disc-shaped electrodes, stacked so that they are orthogonal to the tissue surface. Regional gradients of rate distinguish driver regions (faster sites) from followers. The variability (or lack thereof) distinguishes zones of high circuit core density in multi-wavelet reentry (high variability) from periodic focal rotors.

What do we do about it?

Decreasing the atria's capacity to sustain fibrillation requires *all* drivers to be addressed. Driver elimination demands circuit transection. Focal and moving drivers need different ablation strategies. Focal rotors must be located, and ablation must extend from their core to a boundary. Moving circuits move, so ablation is directed at distributing lines, in order to maximize the probability of meandering cores colliding with boundaries. The optimal distribution of ablation lines is that which achieves these goals *with the fewest ablation lesions*. The most efficient distribution of ablation lesions can be identified based upon

---

[52] Technically, a single moving rotor that conducts 1 : 1 on every beat will generate a changing atrial activation sequence simply by virtue of moving. However, there have been no studies of AF that suggest that a single organized meandering rotor sustains itself for any significant length of time. Multi-focal firing can also generate a changing activation sequence, but this too has not been demonstrated in any ongoing fashion.

[53] So, lots of stuff causes fibrillation.

atrial geometry, knowledge of circuit type(s), and the distribution and preferential directions of core meander. For AF driven only by moving circuits, optimization correlates with the weighted average distance metric (for a given atrial anatomy and circuit distribution). When AF is driven by a mixture of stationary and moving circuits, optimization is achieved with the *constrained*, weighted average distance method; lesion distributions considered in the optimization algorithm must include lines that pass through (or isolate) all stationary circuit cores.[54]

---

[54] There, was that so hard?

Appendix A: Calculating probability in a random walk

Using a simplistic example of a random walk (on a one-dimensional number line), let's examine how we calculate the probability of our walker "hitting a boundary." Let's set the following conditions: the walker starts at 0, takes one step at a time (and cannot remain in place), and flips a "fair" coin to decide whether to go in the forward (positive) or backward (negative) direction with each step. A fair coin has a 50/50 chance of landing on heads. The **probability** of a particular outcome **is related to the number of ways that that outcome could occur, divided by the total possible outcomes**. Thus, if the walker starts at 0 and the boundaries are at −5 and 5, then the probability of hitting a boundary after one time-step is 0 (the walker can only land on −1 or 1; Figure 88, first flip). After the second time-step there are more possibilities; note that where the walker is on the second step depends in part upon where he went in the first step (Figure 88, second flip). If we continue flipping our coin and plotting the possible locations of the walker for 5 flips/steps, we have 32 possible final locations, only two of which are boundaries (−5 and 5). Thus, the probability of "hitting a boundary" in ≤5 steps is 2/32 = 6.25%.

Understanding Atrial Fibrillation, First Edition. Peter Spector.
© 2020 John Wiley & Sons Ltd. Published 2020 by John Wiley & Sons Ltd.

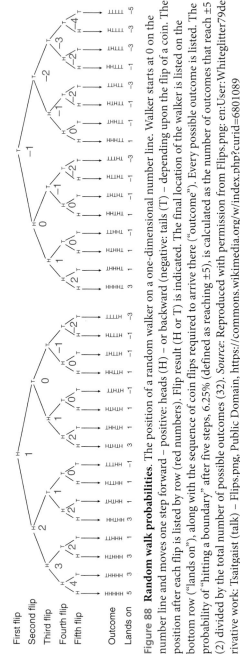

Figure 88 Random walk probabilities. The position of a random walker on a one-dimensional number line. Walker starts at 0 on the number line and moves one step forward – positive: heads (H) – or backward (negative: tails (T) – depending upon the flip of a coin. The position after each flip is listed by row (red numbers). Flip result (H or T) is indicated. The final location of the walker is listed on the bottom row ("lands on"), along with the sequence of coin flips required to arrive there ("outcome"). Every possible outcome is listed. The probability of "hitting a boundary" after five steps, 6.25% (defined as reaching ±5), is calculated as the number of outcomes that reach ±5 (2) divided by the total number of possible outcomes (32). *Source:* Reproduced with permission from Flips.png: en:User:Whiteglitter79de rivative work: Tsaitgaist (talk) – Flips.png, Public Domain, https://commons.wikimedia.org/w/index.php?curid=6801089

Appendix B: Dominant frequency analysis

Because few clinical electrophysiologists are familiar with dominant frequency (DF) analysis, it is hard for us to think critically about studies that make use of DF for mapping atrial fibrillation (AF). Without getting into the details of the math, we can nonetheless get a feel for what DF mapping entails and what its vulnerabilities are. There is an excellent paper that reviews DF mapping for clinicians, which I highly recommend [83]. As mentioned in the main text of this book, frequency domain analysis is an alternative way to examine electrograms (a time domain signal), and is particularly useful when complex signal morphology makes direct interpretation challenging. Frequency domain analysis is based upon the idea that one can "decompose" a time domain signal into a series of sine waves of varied amplitude (and phase). Figure 89

gives a feel for how this works with a square wave (bottom row, middle column). What we see in the figure is that the "dominant frequency" (bottom row, right column) in the power spectrum of the square wave is a sine wave that has the same frequency as the square wave. The other frequencies are required to turn the smooth sinusoidal wave (top left) into a sharp-cornered square wave. The "power" in the power spectrum reflects the amplitude that a particular sine wave contributes to the original signal. Fourier transformation is a mathematical operation performed on *continuous* signals. For discrete signals (e.g. digitized data), we employ the Fast Fourier Transform (FFT). I mention this only because discretization turns this into a sampling problem (see Section 3.1.1). The frequency resolution of the FFT

Understanding Atrial Fibrillation, First Edition. Peter Spector.
© 2020 John Wiley & Sons Ltd. Published 2020 by John Wiley & Sons Ltd.

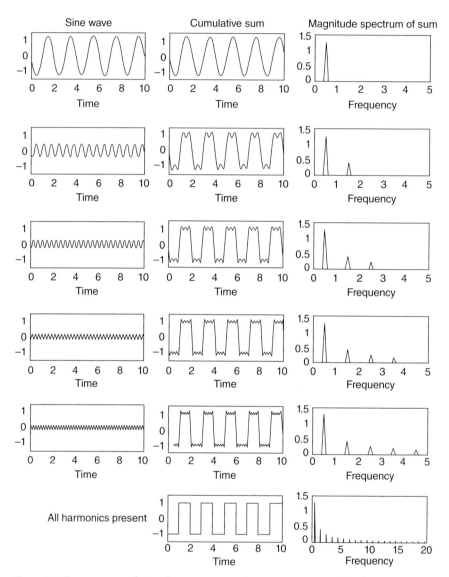

Figure 89 Frequency analysis of a square wave. A square wave signal (middle column, bottom) can be reproduced as the composition of sine waves of various frequencies and amplitudes (left). The signal composed from a cumulative superposition of sine waves is seen (middle top to bottom). The resultant power spectrum at each step is shown (right). As sine waves of higher frequency and lower amplitude are added, the cumulative sum looks more and more like a square wave. *Source*: Reproduced with permission from [83].

is the sample frequency divided by the number of points analyzed. Thus, "Assuming a sampling rate of 1,000 samples per second or 1 kHz, 10-seconds or 10,000 samples of recording are needed to obtain a frequency resolution of 0.1 Hz. There is a tradeoff between the frequency resolution and the time resolution" [83]. In other words, if you analyze a longer recording your frequency resolution is higher (you can distinguish smaller changes in frequency), but you will be blind to any changes in frequency that occur *during* the length of the analyzed recording. When we perform an FFT analysis we extract the frequency content of the signal, but lose all of the timing content within the signal (we don't know *when* a frequency component occurred).

Who cares about any of this? The reason we are going through this exercise is to better understand frequency analysis *of electrograms*: "If the signal is highly periodic and more or less sinusoidal in morphology, the dominant frequency will in most cases be related to the rate of the signal" [83]. AF signals do not particularly fit this description. For starters, they are *not* sinusoidal. Electrograms are sharp and therefore require pre-processing in order to perform FFT analysis (Figure 90), unlike the signals in optical mapping (which are more sinusoidal to begin with). In addition, "Other common properties of AF electrograms, such as high variability of the activation intervals and complex fractionation, unfortunately present as much difficulty for dominant frequency analysis as they do in time domain analysis because the signals are not easily characterized by a sine wave that corresponds to the frequency of activation" (Figure 91) [83]. This is why we felt that using high-resolution electrodes to produce discrete local activation signals would be preferable to FFT analysis.

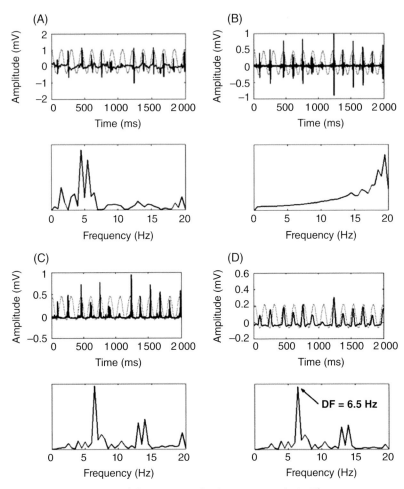

Figure 90 Pre-processing of electrograms for frequency analysis. Electrograms are too sharp to be easily "fit" with sine waves. Therefore pre-processing steps are taken to make the electrograms more rounded. Processing steps and the resultant power spectrum are illustrated: original bipolar signal (A), band-pass filtered signal (40–250 Hz) (B), rectification (C), and low-pass filtering with a 20 Hz cut-off frequency (D). Note that in this example the dominant frequency (DF) changes from <5 Hz in the original signal to 6.5 Hz in the final pre-processed signal. *Source*: Reproduced with permission from [83].

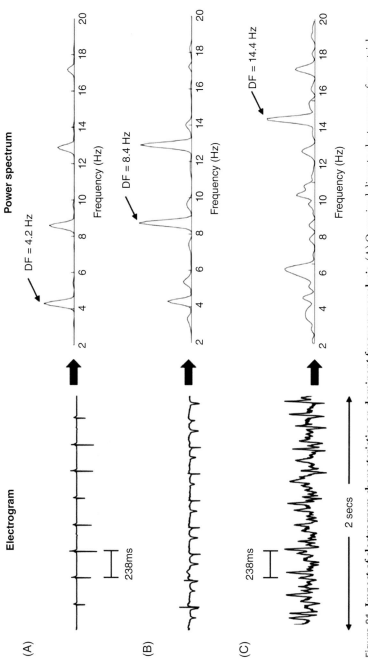

Figure 91 Impact of electrogram characteristics on dominant frequency analysis. (A) Organized discrete electrograms from atrial flutter. Cycle length (238 ms) correlates well with the dominant frequency (DF; 4.2 Hz). (B) A second electrogram recorded during atrial flutter, at a location that has both far-field and near-field signals (same cycle length), but now the DF is 8.4 Hz due to "over-counting," i.e. the rate of deflections is different from the rate of the arrhythmia waves. (C) Electrogram recorded during atrial fibrillation. The DF is 14.4 Hz corresponding to a cycle length of 69 ms, which is unlikely in a human atrium. *Source:* Reproduced with permission from [144].

Appendix C: A stupid idea, but a learning opportunity

When I first started trying to ablate atrial fibrillation (AF), I had the sense that the *only* problem with AF ablation was our inability to map it. I felt sure that if we could "see" AF we would know what was causing it, and that this in turn would lead to an obvious strategy for how to treat it. While I still believe that in order to treat AF we need to identify the location(s) and mechanism(s) of its drivers, I no longer think that simply seeing AF reveals its remedies.

Not long after the idea of finding and eliminating the triggers that initiate AF got everyone started on ablating AF, the idea of dominant frequency (DF) mapping was introduced. Jalife's group had identified the focal drivers of fibrillation and demonstrated that one could discern regional gradients in excitation rates, and that the faster regions were driving the slow regions [41]. One problem with frequency mapping of AF was that it could be very difficult to determine local cycle length using electrograms. All too often electrograms were fractionated. This made it impossible to identify which deflection(s) represented local activation, precluding determination of cycle length (time between successive activations). Instead, based upon Jalife's approach, several papers came out in which investigators examined electrograms in the frequency domain rather than the time domain. This, as we've seen, is a mathematical technique for identifying the underlying excitation rate *without* having to identify local activation time. At the time I didn't understand "fast Fourier transform" (FFT) analysis at all. The *point* of this story relates to what I learned about electrical currents

Understanding Atrial Fibrillation, First Edition. Peter Spector.
© 2020 John Wiley & Sons Ltd. Published 2020 by John Wiley & Sons Ltd.

and electrograms as a result of *not* understanding DF mapping.

I had an inherent skepticism of DF mapping. I felt (due to my ignorance) that it was a black box: input a signal whose cycle length you couldn't discern and output a number. I'm too much of an anti-authoritarian for that sort of thing. I decided to try to teach myself about DF mapping empirically. With the help of people in the college of engineering (I work at a university!), I performed the following, misguided experiments.

First, I "created" a signal with a "known" frequency. I simply made a straight-line signal and introduced a discrete deflection at whatever interval I wanted (Figure 92A). I then performed an FFT on the signal and compared the "accuracy" of the DF result with the "answer," which was the inverse of the actual cycle lengths I had created. I next varied the amplitude of the deflections, the cycle lengths, or both, to see how these things effected the "accuracy"[1] of the DF.

The next thing I did was to use real electrograms and place them in a line of "zeros" (Figure 92) in order to create real-ish electrograms, but ones in which I knew the real cycle length. Finally, I used real electrograms of

varying degrees of complexity/fractionation. Again, I played the "place them on an otherwise straight line" game to generate tracings with whatever frequency I chose, and compared this to the result of the FFT. I managed to "trick" the FFT: it kept getting the wrong answer.[2]

You've probably seen my error right from the start here. (If not, don't feel bad, they made *me* a professor of engineering!) The mistake I was making was in misunderstanding the fundamental question: *frequency of what?* The FFT isn't wrong. It tells you the result of applying some calculations on the signal you feed it. It tells you (as best it can) what various frequencies of sine waves which, when combined, best reproduce that signal. I thought that it was wrong, because I thought that I knew what the "real" frequency was (the inverse of the cycle lengths that I had created). Here's the mistake. I imagined that the FFT was "trying" to identify how often a wave of excitation propagated beneath the electrode. That is *not* what it does. It simply identifies information about the frequency content of the squiggly line you feed it. It doesn't know what generated that signal. The disconnect isn't between the calculated frequency

---

[1] Why I keep using quotations around accuracy will become clear.

[2] I can be very clever when I'm completely missing the point.

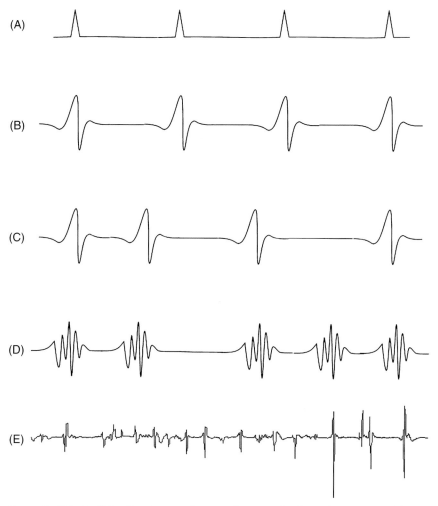

Figure 92 **"Testing" fast Fourier transform analysis**. Artificial signals were created first, with (A) monophasic deflections evenly spaced on a zero baseline. Next, realistic electrograms were evenly spaced (B) or irregularly spaced (C). We created irregularly spaced complex electrograms (D) and real, complex electrograms from clinical recordings (E).

content of the signal and the actual frequency content of the signal; the signal frequency is the signal frequency. The disconnect is between the signal (the electrogram) and the waves of excitation that generate the electrogram. I simply never thought about it. I didn't explicitly think "the electrogram and the waves are the same thing," it was just the *implicit premise* of my thinking about electrograms.

Let's dig a little into my error. I imagined that a complex electrogram (Figure 92), the "chunk" that I placed on a line, was a single thing. How often I placed one of those things on a line determined the frequency of the resultant signal. This was the error. The FFT is determining information about the frequency content with which the line deviates from zero. The reason I made that error is that I was stuck on the idea that the electrogram was equivalent to the wave; one wave goes by the electrode, one electrogram (complex) is inscribed on the tracing. That isn't quite accurate. Whenever currents in the underlying tissue produce perturbations in the potential field at the electrode surface, the signal deviates from baseline. Because currents produce perturbations in the potential field that are measurable for some distance away from the site of the current, there isn't a 1 : 1 relationship between wave and electrogram "complex." The relationship is between wave and *deflection*.[3] Each of multiple independent waves generates a deflection; a complex electrogram can reflect multiple waves, they are not a unit. I was thinking about *coherent* waves. By this I mean a coordinated wave such that the number of times a wave passes a region is equal to the number of times when each cell in that region is excited. During sinus rhythm, the number of cell excitations, number of waves, and number of "electrograms" are all the same.

Imagine an electrode sitting near the end of a linear scar (Figure 93). If the electrode can "see" waves as they pass along *either* side of the scar, one can see a "double" electrogram (Figure 93). In this setting, the number of deflections and the number of times any particular cell is excited is not equal. We are looking at one side and then the other. An easy way to see how we could misinterpret this would be if there were reentry around the scar, and our electrode was in the middle. In this case, we see the wave as it passes up one side and *again* as it passes down the other side of the scar. By placing our electrode in the middle of the scar, the deflections are equally spaced on the tracing. One could now see how it would be easy to misinterpret the rate of reentry: you could easily think it was twice as fast as it actually is.

---

[3] Even this is not quite accurate. If two waves pass near the electrode *at the same time*, they will produce a single deflection (the waves are superimposed). Independent deflections require spatial *and temporal* separation.

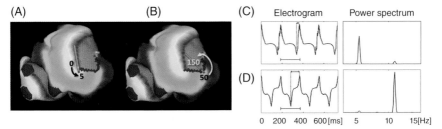

Figure 93 Double potentials and dominant frequency (DF) mapping. Waves on both sides of a linear scar can be seen by an electrode placed near the scar. The potential time farther apart or closer together depends upon the proximity of the electrode to the turnaround point (end of the scar). (A) When the electrode is placed at the edge of the scar it records a single biphasic deflection (C), which generates an "appropriate" DF (equal to the inverse of the tachycardia cycle length). When the electrode is placed along the middle of the scar, such that it records a deflection when the wave passes below *and* above the scar (B), the "biphasic" electrogram is seen as two distinct deflections (D) and the DF "double counts," yielding an "inappropriately" high DF. *Source*: Reproduced with permission from Visible Electrophysiology LLC.

References

1. Spector, P. (2016). *Understanding Clinical Cardiac Electrophysiology: A Conceptually Guided Approach.* Chichester: Wiley.

2. Wu, T.J., Yashima, M., Xie, F. et al. (1998). Role of pectinate muscle bundles in the generation and maintenance of intra-atrial reentry: potential implications for the mechanism of conversion between atrial fibrillation and atrial flutter. *Circ. Res.* **83** (4): 448–462.

3. Filgueiras-Rama, D. and Jalife, J. (2016). Structural and functional bases of cardiac fibrillation. Differences and similarities between atria and ventricles. *JACC Clin. Electrophysiol.* **2** (1): 1–3.

4. Garfinkel, A., Kim, Y.-H., Voroshilovsky, O. et al. (2000). Preventing ventricular fibrillation by flattening cardiac restitution. *Proc. Natl. Acad. Sci. U. S. A.* **97** (11): 6061–6066.

5. Qu, Z., Kil, J., Zie, F. et al. (2000). Scroll wave dynamics in a three-dimensional cardiac tissue model: roles of restitution, thickness, and fiber rotation. *Biophys. J.* **78** (6): 2761–2775.

6. Xie, F., Qu, Z., Garfinkel, A. et al. (2002). Electrical refractory period restitution and spiral wave reentry in simulated cardiac tissue. *Am. J. Physiol. Heart Circ. Physiol.* **283** (1): H448–H460.

7. Narayan, S.M., Kazi, D., Krummen, D.E. et al. (2008). Repolarization and activation restitution near human pulmonary veins and atrial fibrillation initiation: a mechanism for the initiation of atrial fibrillation by premature beats. *J. Am. Coll. Cardiol.* **52** (15): 1222–1230.

8. Franz, M.R. (2003). The electrical restitution curve revisited: steep or flat slope – which is better? *J. Cardiovasc. Electrophysiol.* **14** (10 Suppl): S140–S147.

9. Allessie, M.A., Bonke, F.I., and Schopman, F.J. (1976). Circus movement in rabbit atrial muscle as a mechanism of tachycardia. II. The role of nonuniform recovery of excitability in the occurrence of unidirectional block, as studied with multiple microelectrodes. *Circ. Res.* **39** (2): 168–177.

10. Ikeda, T., Uchida, T., Hough, D. et al. (1996). Mechanism of spontaneous termination of functional reentry in isolated canine right atrium. Evidence for the presence of an excitable but nonexcited core. *Circulation* **94** (8): 1962–1973.

11. McWilliam, J.A. (1887). Fibrillar contraction of the heart. *J. Physiol.* **8** (5): 296–310.

12. Garrey, W. (1924). *Auricular Fibrillation. Physiol. Rev.* **4** (2): 215–250. https://doi.org/10.1152/physrev.1924.4.2.215.

13. Mackenzie, J. (1911). The Schorstein lectures on AURICULAR FIBRILLATION: delivered at the London hospital, October, 1911. *Br. Med. J.* **2** (2650): 869–874.

14. Lewis, T. (1912). A lecture on THE EVIDENCES OF AURICULAR FIBRILLATION, TREATED HISTORICALLY: delivered at University College Hospital. *Br. Med. J.* **1** (2663): 57–60.

15. Mines, G.R. (1913). On dynamic equilibrium in the heart. *J. Physiol.* **46** (4–5): 349–383.

16. Lewis, T., Drury, A.N., Iliescu, C.C. et al. (1921). The manner in which quinidine sulphate acts in auricular fibrillation. *Br. Med. J.* **2** (3170): 514–515.

17. Garrey, W.E. (1914). The nature of fibrillatory contraction of the heart – its relation to tissue mass and form. *Am. J. Phys.* **33**: 397–414.

18. Moe, G.K. and Abildskov, J.A. (1959). Atrial fibrillation as a self-sustaining arrhythmia independent of focal discharge. *Am. Heart J.* **58** (1): 59–70.

19. Moe, G.K., Rheinboldt, W.C., and Abildskov, J.A. (1964). A computer model of atrial fibrillation. *Am. Heart J.* **67**: 200–220.

20. Konings, K.T., Kirchhof, C.J., Smeets, J.R. et al. (1994). High-density mapping of electrically induced atrial fibrillation in humans. *Circulation* **89** (4): 1665–1680.

21. Janse, M.J., Wilms-Schopman, F.J., and Coronel, R. (1995). Ventricular fibrillation is not always due to multiple wavelet reentry. *J. Cardiovasc. Electrophysiol.* **6** (7): 512–521.

22. Chen, P.S., Garfinkel, A., Weiss, J.N. et al. (1998). Computerized mapping of fibrillation in normal ventricular myocardium. *Chaos* **8** (1): 127–136.

23. Cox, J.L., Canavan, T.E., Schuessler, R.B. et al. (1991). The surgical treatment of atrial fibrillation. II. Intraoperative electrophysiologic mapping and description of the electrophysiologic basis of atrial flutter and atrial fibrillation. *J. Thorac. Cardiovasc. Surg.* **101** (3): 406–426.

24. Cox, J.L. (2011). The first Maze procedure. *J. Thorac. Cardiovasc. Surg.* **141** (5): 1093–1097.

25. Prasad, S.M., Maniar, H.S., Camillo, C.J. et al. (2003). The Cox maze III procedure for atrial fibrillation: long-term efficacy in patients undergoing lone versus concomitant procedures. *J. Thorac. Cardiovasc. Surg.* **126** (6): 1822–1828.

26. Damiano, R.J. Jr., Schwartz, F.H., Bailey, M.S. et al. (2011). The Cox maze IV procedure: predictors of late recurrence. *J. Thorac. Cardiovasc. Surg.* **141** (1): 113–121.

27. Ikeda, T., Yashima, M., Uchida, T. et al. (1997). Attachment of meandering reentrant wave fronts to anatomic obstacles in the atrium. Role of the obstacle size. *Circ. Res.* **81** (5): 753–764.

28. Filgueiras-Rama, D., Martins, R.P., Mironov, S. et al. (2012). Chloroquine terminates stretch-induced atrial fibrillation more effectively than flecainide in the sheep heart. *Circ. Arrhythm. Electrophysiol.* **5** (3): 561–570.

29. Pandit, S.V., Zlochiver, S., Filgueiras-Rama, D. et al. (2011). Targeting atrioventricular differences in ion channel properties for terminating acute atrial fibrillation in pigs. *Cardiovasc. Res.* **89** (4): 843–851.

30. Davidenko, J.M., Pertsov, A.V., Salomonsz, R. et al. (1992). Stationary and drifting spiral waves of excitation in isolated cardiac muscle. *Nature* **355** (6358): 349–351.

31. Pandit, S.V., Berenfeld, O., Anumonwo, J.M. et al. (2005). Ionic determinants of functional reentry in a 2-D model of human atrial cells during simulated chronic atrial fibrillation. *Biophys. J.* **88** (6): 3806–3821.

32. Asano, Y., Saito, J., Matsumoto, K. et al. (1992). On the mechanism of termination and perpetuation of atrial fibrillation. *Am. J. Cardiol.* **69** (12): 1033–1038.

33. Rensma, P.L., Allessie, M.A., Lammers, W.J. et al. (1988). Length of excitation wave and susceptibility to reentrant atrial arrhythmias in normal conscious dogs. *Circ. Res.* **62** (2): 395–410.

34. Carrick, R.T., Bates, O.R., Benson, B.E. et al. (2015). Prospectively quantifying the propensity for atrial fibrillation: a mechanistic formulation. *PLoS One* **10** (3): e0118746.

35. Rappel, W.J., Zaman, J.A., and Narayan, S.M. (2015). Mechanisms for the termination of atrial fibrillation by localized ablation: computational and clinical studies. *Circ. Arrhythm. Electrophysiol.* **8** (6): 1325–1333.

36. Carrick, R.T., Benson, B.E., Bates, J.H. et al. (2016). Prospective, tissue-specific optimization of ablation for multiwavelet reentry: predicting the required amount, location, and configuration of lesions. *Circ. Arrhythm. Electrophysiol.* **9** (3): pii: e003555.

37. Scherf, D., Romano, F.J., and Terranova, R. (1948). Experimental studies on auricular flutter and auricular fibrillation. *Am. Heart J.* **36** (2): 241–251.

38. Davidenko, J.M., Kent, P.F., Chialvo, D.R. et al. (1990). Sustained vortex-like waves in normal isolated ventricular muscle. *Proc. Natl. Acad. Sci. U. S. A.* **87** (22): 8785–8789.

39. Pertsov, A.M., Davidenko, J.M., Salomonsz, R. et al. (1993). Spiral waves of excitation underlie reentrant activity in isolated cardiac muscle. *Circ. Res.* **72** (3): 631–650.

40. Gray, R.A., Pertsov, A.M., and Jalife, J. (1998). Spatial and temporal organization during cardiac fibrillation. *Nature* **392** (6671): 75–78.

41. Skanes, A.C., Mandapati, R., Berenfeld, O. et al. (1998). Spatiotemporal periodicity during atrial

fibrillation in the isolated sheep heart. *Circulation* **98** (12): 1236–1248.

42. Mandapati, R., Skanes, A., Chen, J. et al. (2000). Stable microreentrant sources as a mechanism of atrial fibrillation in the isolated sheep heart. *Circulation* **101** (2): 194–199.

43. Zou, R., Kneller, J., Leon, L.J. et al. (2005). Substrate size as a determinant of fibrillatory activity maintenance in a mathematical model of canine atrium. *Am. J. Physiol. Heart Circ. Physiol.* **289** (3): H1002–H1012.

44. Hansen, B.J., Zhao, J., Csepe, T.A. et al. (2015). Atrial fibrillation driven by micro-anatomic intramural re-entry revealed by simultaneous sub-epicardial and sub-endocardial optical mapping in explanted human hearts. *Eur. Heart J.* **36** (35): 2390–2401.

45. Zhao, J., Hansen, B.J., Wang, Y. et al. (2017). Three-dimensional integrated functional, structural, and computational mapping to define the structural "fingerprints" of heart-specific atrial fibrillation drivers in human heart ex vivo. *J. Am. Heart Assoc.* **6** (8): pii: e005922.

46. Schuessler, R.B., Kawamoto, T., Hand, D.E. et al. (1993). Simultaneous epicardial and endocardial activation sequence mapping in the isolated canine right atrium. *Circulation* **88** (1): 250–263.

47. Eckstein, J., Maesen, B., Linz, D. et al. (2011). Time course and mechanisms of endo-epicardial electrical dissociation during atrial fibrillation in the goat. *Cardiovasc. Res.* **89** (4): 816–824.

48. Verheule, S., Eckstein, J., Linz, D. et al. (2014). Role of endo-epicardial dissociation of electrical activity and transmural conduction in the development of persistent atrial fibrillation. *Prog. Biophys. Mol. Biol.* **115** (2–3): 173–185.

49. Allessie, M.A., de Groot, N.M., Houben, R.P. et al. (2010). Electropathological substrate of long-standing persistent atrial fibrillation in patients with structural heart disease: longitudinal dissociation. *Circ. Arrhythm. Electrophysiol.* **3** (6): 606–615.

50. de Groot, N.M., Houben, R.P., Smeets, J.L. et al. (2010). Electropathological substrate of longstanding persistent atrial fibrillation in patients with structural heart disease: epicardial breakthrough. *Circulation* **122** (17): 1674–1682.

51. de Groot, N., van der Does, L., Yaksh, A. et al. (2016). Direct proof of endo-epicardial asynchrony of the atrial wall during atrial fibrillation in humans. *Circ. Arrhythm. Electrophysiol.* **9** (5): pii: e003648.

52. Tanaka, K., Zlochiver, S., Vikstrom, K.L. et al. (2007). Spatial distribution of fibrosis governs fibrillation wave dynamics in the posterior left atrium during heart failure. *Circ. Res.* **101** (8): 839–847.

53. Lee, G., Kumar, S., The, A. et al. (2014). Epicardial wave mapping in human long-lasting persistent atrial fibrillation: transient rotational circuits, complex wavefronts, and disorganized activity. *Eur. Heart J.* **35** (2): 86–97.

54. Chen, J., Mandapati, R., Berenfeld, O. et al. (2000). Dynamics of wavelets

and their role in atrial fibrillation in the isolated sheep heart. *Cardiovasc. Res.* **48** (2): 220–232.

55. Fareh, S., Villemaire, C., and Nattel, S. (1998). Importance of refractoriness heterogeneity in the enhanced vulnerability to atrial fibrillation induction caused by tachycardia-induced atrial electrical remodeling. *Circulation* **98** (20): 2202–2209.

56. Ogawa, M., Kumagai, K., Gondo, N. et al. (2002). Novel electrophysiologic parameter of dispersion of atrial repolarization: comparison of different atrial pacing methods. *J. Cardiovasc. Electrophysiol.* **13** (2): 110–117.

57. Oliveira, M.M., da Silva, N., Timóteo, A.T. et al. (2007). Enhanced dispersion of atrial refractoriness as an electrophysiological substrate for vulnerability to atrial fibrillation in patients with paroxysmal atrial fibrillation. *Rev. Port. Cardiol.* **26** (7–8): 691–702.

58. Schuessler, R.B., Kay, M.W., Melby, S.J. et al. (2006). Spatial and temporal stability of the dominant frequency of activation in human atrial fibrillation. *J. Electrocardiol.* **39** (4 Suppl): S7–S12.

59. Atienza, F., Almendral, J., Jalife, J. et al. (2009). Real-time dominant frequency mapping and ablation of dominant frequency sites in atrial fibrillation with left-to-right frequency gradients predicts long-term maintenance of sinus rhythm. *Heart Rhythm.* **6** (1): 33–40.

60. Jarman, J.W., Wong, T., Kojodjojo, P. et al. (2012). Spatiotemporal behavior of high dominant frequency during paroxysmal and persistent atrial fibrillation in the human left atrium. *Circ. Arrhythm. Electrophysiol.* **5** (4): 650–658.

61. Montenero, A.S., Franciosa, P., Mangiameli, D. et al. (2001). Different atrial regional patterns of activation during atrial fibrillation: is there any relationship with the anatomy? *Ann. Ist. Super. Sanita.* **37** (3): 429–434.

62. Cha, T.J., Ehrlich, J.R., Zhang, L. et al. (2005). Atrial tachycardia remodeling of pulmonary vein cardiomyocytes: comparison with left atrium and potential relation to arrhythmogenesis. *Circulation* **111** (6): 728–735.

63. Filgueiras-Rama, D., Martins, R.P., Ennis, S.R. et al. (2011). High-resolution endocardial and epicardial optical mapping in a sheep model of stretch-induced atrial fibrillation. *J. Vis. Exp.* **53**: pii: 3103.

64. Skanes, A.C., Gray, R.A., Zuur, C.L. et al. (1997). Spatio-temporal patterns of atrial fibrillation: role of the subendocardial structure. *Semin. Interv. Cardiol.* **2** (4): 185–193.

65. Wieser, L., Fischer, G., Nowak, C.N. et al. (2007). Fibrillatory conduction in branching atrial tissue – insight from volumetric and monolayer computer models. *Comput. Methods Prog. Biomed.* **86** (2): 103–111.

66. Gonzales, M.J., Vincent, K.P., Rappel, W.J. et al. (2014). Structural contributions to fibrillatory rotors in a patient-derived computational model of the atria. *Europace* **16** (Suppl 4): iv3–iv10.

67. Haissaguerre, M., Shah, A.J., Cochet, H. et al. (2016). Intermittent drivers anchoring to structural heterogeneities as a major pathophysiological mechanism of human persistent atrial fibrillation. *J. Physiol.* **594** (9): 2387–2398.

68. Warren, M., Guha, P.K., Berenfeld, O. et al. (2003). Blockade of the inward rectifying potassium current terminates ventricular fibrillation in the guinea pig heart. *J. Cardiovasc. Electrophysiol.* **14** (6): 621–631.

69. Voigt, N., Trausch, A., Knaut, M. et al. (2010). Left-to-right atrial inward rectifier potassium current gradients in patients with paroxysmal versus chronic atrial fibrillation. *Circ. Arrhythm. Electrophysiol.* **3** (5): 472–480.

70. Walters, T.E., Lee, G., Morris, G. et al. (2015). Temporal stability of rotors and atrial activation patterns in persistent human atrial fibrillation: a high-density epicardial mapping study of prolonged recordings. *JACC Clin. Electrophysiol.* **1** (1–2): 14–24.

71. Campbell, K., Calvo, C.J., Mironov, S. et al. (2012). Spatial gradients in action potential duration created by regional magnetofection of hERG are a substrate for wavebreak and turbulent propagation in cardiomyocyte monolayers. *J. Physiol.* **590** (24): 6363–6379.

72. Sanders, P., Berenfeld, O., Hocini, M. et al. (2005). Spectral analysis identifies sites of high-frequency activity maintaining atrial fibrillation in humans. *Circulation* **112** (6): 789–797.

73. Tobon, C., Rodriguez, J., Ferrero, J. et al. (2012). Dominant frequency and organization index maps in a realistic three-dimensional computational model of atrial fibrillation. *Europace* **14** (Suppl 5): v25–v32.

74. Uldry, L., Virag, N., Kappenberger, L. et al. (2009). Optimization of antitachycardia pacing protocols applied to atrial fibrillation: insights from a biophysical model. *Conf. Proc. IEEE Eng. Med. Biol. Soc.* **2009**: 3024–3027.

75. Noujaim, S.F., Stuckey, J.A., Ponce-Balbuena, D. et al. (2010). Specific residues of the cytoplasmic domains of cardiac inward rectifier potassium channels are effective antifibrillatory targets. *FASEB J.* **24** (11): 4302–4312.

76. Samie, F.H., Berenfeld, O., Anumonwo, J. et al. (2001). Rectification of the background potassium current: a determinant of rotor dynamics in ventricular fibrillation. *Circ. Res.* **89** (12): 1216–1223.

77. Martins, R.P., Kaur, K., Hwang, E. et al. (2014). Dominant frequency increase rate predicts transition from paroxysmal to long-term persistent atrial fibrillation. *Circulation* **129** (14): 1472–1482.

78. Ehrlich, J.R., Cha, T.J., Zhang, L. et al. (2003). Cellular electrophysiology of canine pulmonary vein cardiomyocytes: action potential and ionic current properties. *J. Physiol.* **551** (Pt 3): 801–813.

79. Calvo, C.J., Deo, M., Zlochiver, S. et al. (2014). Attraction of rotors to the pulmonary veins in paroxysmal atrial fibrillation: a modeling study. *Biophys. J.* **106** (8): 1811–1821.

80. Ashihara, T., Namba, T., Ito, M. et al. (2004). Spiral wave control by a localized stimulus: a bidomain model study. *J. Cardiovasc. Electrophysiol.* **15** (2): 226–233.

81. Yamazaki, M., Vaquero, L.M., Hou, L. et al. (2009). Mechanisms of stretch-induced atrial fibrillation in the presence and the absence of adrenocholinergic stimulation: interplay between rotors and focal discharges. *Heart Rhythm.* **6** (7): 1009–1017.

82. Carrick, R.T., Benson, B., Habel, N. et al. (2013). Ablation of multiwavelet re-entry guided by circuit-density and distribution: maximizing the probability of circuit annihilation. *Circ. Arrhythm. Electrophysiol.* **6** (6): 1229–1235.

83. Ng, J. and Goldberger, J.J. (2007). Understanding and interpreting dominant frequency analysis of AF electrograms. *J. Cardiovasc. Electrophysiol.* **18** (6): 680–685.

84. Spach, M.S. and Dolber, P.C. (1986). Relating extracellular potentials and their derivatives to anisotropic propagation at a microscopic level in human cardiac muscle. Evidence for electrical uncoupling of side-to-side fiber connections with increasing age. *Circ. Res.* **58** (3): 356–371.

85. Kalifa, J., Tanaka, K., Zaitsev, A.V. et al. (2006). Mechanisms of wave fractionation at boundaries of high-frequency excitation in the posterior left atrium of the isolated sheep heart during atrial fibrillation. *Circulation* **113** (5): 626–633.

86. Nademanee, K., McKenzie, J., Kosar, E. et al. (2004). A new approach for catheter ablation of atrial fibrillation: mapping of the electrophysiologic substrate. *J. Am. Coll. Cardiol.* **43** (11): 2044–2053.

87. Elayi, C.S., di Biase, L., Bai, R. et al. (2011). Identifying the relationship between the non-PV triggers and the critical CFAE sites post-PVAI to curtail the extent of atrial ablation in longstanding persistent AF. *J. Cardiovasc. Electrophysiol.* **22** (11): 1199–1205.

88. Nademanee, K., Lockwood, E., Oketani, N. et al. Catheter ablation of atrial fibrillation guided by complex fractionated atrial electrogram mapping of atrial fibrillation substrate. *J. Cardiol.* **55** (1): 1–12.

89. Nademanee, K., Schwab, M., Porath, J. et al. (2006). How to perform electrogram-guided atrial fibrillation ablation. *Heart Rhythm.* **3** (8): 981–984.

90. Lesh, M.D., Spear, J.F., and Simson, M.B. (1988). A computer model of the electrogram: what causes fractionation? *J. Electrocardiol.* **21** (Suppl): S69–S73.

91. Umapathy, K., Masse, S., Kolodziejska, K. et al. (2008). Electrogram fractionation in murine HL-1 atrial monolayer model. *Heart Rhythm.* **5** (7): 1029–1035.

92. Gardner, P.I., Ursell, P.C., Fenoglio, J.J. Jr. et al. (1985). Electrophysiologic and anatomic basis for fractionated electrograms recorded from healed myocardial infarcts. *Circulation* **72** (3): 596–611.

93. de Bakker, J.M., van Capelle, F.J., Janse, M.J. et al. (1993). Slow conduction in the infarcted human heart. "Zigzag" course of activation. *Circulation* **88** (3): 915–926.

94. Jacquemet, V. and Henriquez, C.S. (2009). Genesis of complex fractionated atrial electrograms in zones of slow conduction: a computer model of microfibrosis. *Heart Rhythm.* **6** (6): 803–810.

95. Zlochiver, S., Yamazaki, M., Kalifa, J. et al. (2008). Rotor meandering contributes to irregularity in electrograms during atrial fibrillation. *Heart Rhythm.* **5** (6): 846–854.

96. Correa de Sa, D.D., Thompson, N., Stinnett-Donnelly, J. et al. (2011). Electrogram fractionation: the relationship between spatiotemporal variation of tissue excitation and electrode spatial resolution. *Circ. Arrhythm. Electrophysiol.* **4** (6): 909–916.

97. Berenfeld, O., Ennis, S., Hwang, E. et al. (2011). Time- and frequency-domain analyses of atrial fibrillation activation rate: the optical mapping reference. *Heart Rhythm.* **8** (11): 1758–1765.

98. Benson, B.E., Carrick, R., Habel, N. et al. (2014). Mapping multi-wavelet reentry without isochrones: an electrogram-guided approach to define substrate distribution. *Europace* **16** (suppl 4): iv102–iv109.

99. Stinnett-Donnelly, J.M., Thompson, N., Habel, N. et al. (2012). Effects of electrode size and spacing on the resolution of intracardiac electrograms. *Coron. Artery Dis.* **23** (2): 126–132.

100. Thompson, N.C., Stinnett-Donnelly, J., Habel, N. et al. (2014). Improved spatial resolution and electrogram wave direction independence with the use of an orthogonal electrode configuration. *J. Clin. Monit. Comput.* **28** (2): 157–163.

101. Konings, K.T., Smeets, J.L., Penn, O.C. et al. (1997). Configuration of unipolar atrial electrograms during electrically induced atrial fibrillation in humans. *Circulation* **95** (5): 1231–1241.

102. Verma, A., Novak, P., Macle, L. et al. (2008). A prospective, multicenter evaluation of ablating complex fractionated electrograms (CFEs) during atrial fibrillation (AF) identified by an automated mapping algorithm: acute effects on AF and efficacy as an adjuvant strategy. *Heart Rhythm.* **5** (2): 198–205.

103. Lin, Y.J., Tai, C.-T., Chang, S.-L. et al. (2009). Efficacy of additional ablation of complex fractionated atrial electrograms for catheter ablation of nonparoxysmal atrial fibrillation. *J. Cardiovasc. Electrophysiol.* **20** (6): 607–615.

104. Li, W.J., Bai, Y.Y., Zhang, H.Y. et al. (2011). Additional ablation of complex fractionated atrial electrograms after pulmonary vein isolation in patients with atrial fibrillation: a meta-analysis. *Circ. Arrhythm. Electrophysiol.* **4** (2): 143–148.

105. Kumagai, K., Nakano, M., Kutsuzawa, D. et al. (2016). The efficacy of ablation based on the combined use of the dominant frequency and complex fractionated atrial

electrograms for non-paroxysmal atrial fibrillation. *J. Cardiol.* **67** (6): 545–550.

106. Ammar-Busch, S., Bourier, F., Reents, T. et al. (2017). Ablation of complex fractionated electrograms with or without ADditional LINEar lesions for persistent atrial fibrillation (the ADLINE trial). *J. Cardiovasc. Electrophysiol.* **28** (6): 636–641.

107. Martin, C.A., Curtain, J.P., Gajendragadkar, P.R. et al. (2018). Ablation of complex fractionated electrograms improves outcome in persistent atrial fibrillation of over 2 year's duration. *J. Atr. Fibrillation* **10** (5): 1607.

108. Oral, H., Chugh, A., Good, E. et al. (2008). Randomized evaluation of right atrial ablation after left atrial ablation of complex fractionated atrial electrograms for long-lasting persistent atrial fibrillation. *Circ. Arrhythm. Electrophysiol.* **1** (1): 6–13.

109. Khaykin, Y., Skanes, A., Champagne, J. et al. (2009). A randomized controlled trial of the efficacy and safety of electroanatomic circumferential pulmonary vein ablation supplemented by ablation of complex fractionated atrial electrograms versus potential-guided pulmonary vein antrum isolation guided by intracardiac ultrasound. *Circ. Arrhythm. Electrophysiol.* **2** (5): 481–487.

110. Fadahunsi, O., Talabi, T., Olowoyeye, A. et al. (2016). Ablation of complex fractionated atrial electrograms for atrial fibrillation rhythm control: a systematic review and meta-analysis. *Can. J. Cardiol.* **32** (6): 791–802.

111. Qin, M., Liu, X., Wu, S.-H. et al. (2016). Atrial substrate modification in atrial fibrillation: targeting GP or CFAE? Evidence from meta-analysis of clinical trials. *PLoS One* **11** (10): e0164989.

112. Salinet, J.L., Tuan, J., Salinet, A.S.M. et al. (2014). Distinctive patterns of dominant frequency trajectory behavior in drug-refractory persistent atrial fibrillation: preliminary characterization of spatiotemporal instability. *J. Cardiovasc. Electrophysiol.* **25** (4): 371–379.

113. Habel, N., Znojkiewicz, P., Thompson, N. et al. (2010). The temporal variability of dominant frequency and complex fractionated atrial electrograms constrains the validity of sequential mapping in human atrial fibrillation. *Heart Rhythm.* **7** (5): 586–593.

114. Verma, A., Lakkireddy, D., Wulffhart, Z. et al. (2011). Relationship between complex fractionated electrograms (CFE) and dominant frequency (DF) sites and prospective assessment of adding DF-guided ablation to pulmonary vein isolation in persistent atrial fibrillation (AF). *J. Cardiovasc. Electrophysiol.* **22** (12): 1309–1316.

115. Platonov, P.G., Mitrofanova, L.B., Orshanskaya, V. et al. (2011). Structural abnormalities in atrial walls are associated with presence and persistency of atrial fibrillation but not with age. *J. Am. Coll. Cardiol.* **58** (21): 2225–2232.

116. Hansen, B.J., Zhao, J., and Fedorov, V.V. (2017). Fibrosis and atrial fibrillation: computerized and optical mapping; a view into the human atria at submillimeter resolution. *JACC Clin. Electrophysiol.* **3** (6): 531–546.

117. Vigmond, E., Pashaei, A., Amraoui, S. et al. (2016). Percolation as a mechanism to explain atrial fractionated electrograms and reentry in a fibrosis model based on imaging data. *Heart Rhythm.* **13** (7): 1536–1543.

118. Alonso, S. and Bar, M. (2013). Reentry near the percolation threshold in a heterogeneous discrete model for cardiac tissue. *Phys. Rev. Lett.* **110** (15): 158101.

119. Steinberg, B.E., Glass, L., Shrier, A. et al. (2006). The role of heterogeneities and intercellular coupling in wave propagation in cardiac tissue. *Philos. Trans. A Math. Phys. Eng. Sci.* **364** (1842): 1299–1311.

120. Takemoto, Y., Takanari, H., Honjo, H. et al. (2012). Inhibition of intercellular coupling stabilizes spiral-wave reentry, whereas enhancement of the coupling destabilizes the reentry in favor of early termination. *Am. J. Physiol. Heart Circ. Physiol.* **303** (5): H578–H586.

121. Morgan, R., Colman, M.A., Chubb, H. et al. (2016). Slow conduction in the border zones of patchy fibrosis stabilizes the drivers for atrial fibrillation: insights from multi-scale human atrial modeling. *Front. Physiol.* **7**: 474.

122. Marrouche, N.F., Wilber, D., Hindricks, G. et al. (2014). Association of atrial tissue fibrosis identified by delayed enhancement MRI and atrial fibrillation catheter ablation: the DECAAF study. *JAMA* **311** (5): 498–506.

123. Spragg, D.D., Khurram, I., Zimmerman, S.L. et al. (2012). Initial experience with magnetic resonance imaging of atrial scar and co-registration with electroanatomic voltage mapping during atrial fibrillation: success and limitations. *Heart Rhythm.* **9** (12): 2003–2009.

124. Teh, A.W., Kistler, P.M., Lee, G. et al. (2011). The relationship between complex fractionated electrograms and atrial low-voltage zones during atrial fibrillation and paced rhythm. *Europace* **13** (12): 1709–1716.

125. Ghoraani, B., Dalvi, R., Gizurarson, S. et al. (2013). Localized rotational activation in the left atrium during human atrial fibrillation: relationship to complex fractionated atrial electrograms and low-voltage zones. *Heart Rhythm.* **10** (12): 1830–1838.

126. Schade, A., Nentwich, K., Costello-Boerrigter, L.C. et al. (2016). Spatial relationship of focal impulses, rotors and low voltage zones in patients with persistent atrial fibrillation. *J. Cardiovasc. Electrophysiol.* **27** (5): 507–514.

127. Rolf, S., Kircher, S., Arya, A. et al. (2014). Tailored atrial substrate modification based on low-voltage areas in catheter ablation of atrial fibrillation. *Circ. Arrhythm. Electrophysiol.* **7** (5): 825–833.

128. Kottkamp, H., Berg, J., Bender, R. et al. (2016). Box isolation of fibrotic

areas (BIFA): a patient-tailored substrate modification approach for ablation of atrial fibrillation. *J. Cardiovasc. Electrophysiol.* **27** (1): 22–30.

129. Cutler, M.J., Johnson, J., Abozguia, K. et al. (2016). Impact of voltage mapping to guide whether to perform ablation of the posterior wall in patients with persistent atrial fibrillation. *J. Cardiovasc. Electrophysiol.* **27** (1): 13–21.

130. Jadidi, A.S., Lehrmann, H., Keyl, C. et al. (2016). Ablation of persistent atrial fibrillation targeting low-voltage areas with selective activation characteristics. *Circ. Arrhythm. Electrophysiol.* **9** (3): pii: e002962.

131. Yagishita, A., de Oliveira, S., Cakulev, I. et al. (2016). Correlation of left atrial voltage distribution between sinus rhythm and atrial fibrillation: identifying structural remodeling by 3-D electroanatomic mapping irrespective of the rhythm. *J. Cardiovasc. Electrophysiol.* **27** (8): 905–912.

132. Blandino, A., Bianchi, F., Grossi, S. et al. (2017). Left atrial substrate modification targeting low-voltage areas for catheter ablation of atrial fibrillation: a systematic review and meta-analysis. *Pacing Clin. Electrophysiol.* **40** (2): 199–212.

133. Yagishita, A., Gimbel, J.R., de Oliveira, S. et al. (2017). Long-term outcome of left atrial voltage-guided substrate ablation during atrial fibrillation: a novel adjunctive ablation strategy. *J. Cardiovasc. Electrophysiol.* **28** (2): 147–155.

134. Narayan, S.M., Krummen, D.E., Shivkumar, K. et al. (2012). Treatment of atrial fibrillation by the ablation of localized sources: CONFIRM (conventional ablation for atrial fibrillation with or without focal impulse and rotor modulation) trial. *J. Am. Coll. Cardiol.* **60** (7): 628–636.

135. Shivkumar, K., Ellenbogen, K.A., Hummel, J.D. et al. (2012). Acute termination of human atrial fibrillation by identification and catheter ablation of localized rotors and sources: first multicenter experience of focal impulse and rotor modulation (FIRM) ablation. *J. Cardiovasc. Electrophysiol.* **23** (12): 1277–1285.

136. Buch, E., Share, M., Tung, R. et al. (2016). Long-term clinical outcomes of focal impulse and rotor modulation for treatment of atrial fibrillation: a multicenter experience. *Heart Rhythm.* **13** (3): 636–641.

137. Mohanty, S., Gianni, C., Mohanty, P. et al. (2016). Impact of rotor ablation in nonparoxysmal atrial fibrillation patients: results from the randomized OASIS trial. *J. Am. Coll. Cardiol.* **68** (3): 274–282.

138. Mohanty, S., Mohanty, P., Trivedi, C. et al. (2018). Long-term outcome of pulmonary vein isolation with and without focal impulse and rotor modulation mapping: insights from a meta-analysis. *Circ. Arrhythm. Electrophysiol.* **11** (3): e005789.

139. Schuessler, R.B., Grayson, T.M., Bromberg, B. et al. (1992). Cholinergically mediated tachyarrhythmias

induced by a single extrastimulus in the isolated canine right atrium. *Circ. Res.* **71** (5): 1254–1267.

140. Kneller, J., Zou, R., Vigmond, E.J. et al. (2002). Cholinergic atrial fibrillation in a computer model of a two-dimensional sheet of canine atrial cells with realistic ionic properties. *Circ. Res.* **90** (9): E73–E87.

141. Calkins, H., Reynolds, M.R., Spector, P. et al. (2009). Treatment of atrial fibrillation with antiarrhythmic drugs or radiofrequency ablation: two systematic literature reviews and meta-analyses. *Circ. Arrhythm. Electrophysiol.* **2** (4): 349–361.

142. Spector, P.S., Noori, A.M., Hardin, N.J. et al. (2006). Pulmonary vein encircling ablation alters the atrial electrophysiologic response to autonomic stimulation. *J. Interv. Card. Electrophysiol.* **17** (2): 119–125.

143. Ng, J. and Goldberger, J.J. (2011). Time- and frequency-domain analysis of AF electrograms: simple approaches to a complex arrhythmia? *Heart Rhythm.* **8** (11): 1766–1768.

Index

Note: Page numbers in *italic* refer to figures.

Understanding Atrial Fibrillation, First Edition. Peter Spector.
© 2020 John Wiley & Sons Ltd. Published 2020 by John Wiley & Sons Ltd.